My Simple Changes

Changes

I Healed My Autoimmune Disease and This Is My Story of How.

Brandon Godsey

ISBN: 978-1-7337840-0-9
Library of Congress Control Number: 2019902524

This book is not intended as a substitute for the medical advice of physicians. The reader
should regularly consult a physician in matters relating to his/her health and particularly with
respect to any symptoms that may require diagnosis or medical attention.

Book design by Jeff Merza
Front cover image by Erik Fischer Photography
Back cover image by Dana Patrick
Editing by Meredith Thomas

Printed by California Green Press, Californiagreenpress.com

First printing edition 2019

www.MySimpleChanges.com

My good friend, Cesar Eudave. Thank you for your generosity, friendship and your values.

Also, I couldn't have made it to this point without two main people. Their support, patience, guidance, laughter and love are why I'm still alive. From breaking my arm, through Crohn's disease and My Simple Changes, you've stayed by my side.

Thank you, Mom and Dad.

Table of Contents

INTRODUCTION

In order to understand what we're doing, we need to understand what's being done and what has been done.

The fact is, people living in advanced civilizations contain a third less bacteria in their bodies than generations ago, and a third less than present-day undeveloped nations. Why? Because we're afraid of bacteria. We live too clean. We're exposed to too much. We breathe industrialization. Over the course of the last several decades we've depleted the number of good bacteria in our bodies through food manufacturing, poor nutrition, antibiotics, preventatives, practices, and chemicals.

The evolution of man, and of food.

We've created environments and conditions that allow diseases and ailments to thrive and grow in our exposed bodies. Bodies are being filled with more bad bacteria than good, acidities are unbalanced, enzymes are depleted, and eventually the immune system attacks itself because of the chaos. And we get autoimmune disease. In America alone, over 50 million people have an autoimmune disorder. That's roughly one in every six people in the United States of America suffering from an immune system that attacks itself, causes inflammation, and results in disease or ailments. And the numbers are increasing.

What I've done in the years since my "1 last treatment" is heal myself through food and lifestyle changes, both equally important and simply worked into my busy life. You can do the same. The hardest part? Understanding that it takes time. My story is for you. For proof that it can be done with patience and trust in yourself. The methods I've developed will help you build back the good bacteria, heal the inflammation, balance the gut and microbiome, and leave you with a new set of habits to properly defend yourself against a system built for our consumption—not our healthy consumption—and one that cares very little about...you. Sad, I know. It's nobody's fault. It's just how we've evolved through free enterprise and regulation. But now we're awake, and you can start making changes today.

This book tells my story but also gives you tips, insights, facts, and tools for living healthily in the modern world instead of continuing to struggle to survive. It provides a system built with your best interests in mind. Did you know that 80 percent of the immune system works through the gut? To heal from autoimmune disease, you need to heal your gut. The fact that you're holding this book means you know you need to make changes to the way you're living in order to heal, but where do you start? This book tells you where, and how. This book tells you how to heal and survive in today's world, while still staying true to you.

My understanding didn't come from a book or a university program. It came from decades of personal experience and struggle with a beaten, diseased, and operated-on body. It came from years of obsession with figuring it out to achieving positive results, connecting the knowledge absorbed over thirty years as both patient and practitioner, and finally putting My Simple Changes here. For you. So you can not only live as happily and healthily as possible now, but your future self can be smiling as well. So you can live more days, with the ones you love, doing the things you love.

CHAPTER 1: One Last Treatment

September 4, 2014

152 pounds. 120 minutes. 2 months. 1 last treatment.

In the land of no seasons, 300 days of sunshine, and endless traffic, the Southern California morning brought a fall-filled crisp to the air. Wind and rain from the previous day dissipated the smog that normally weighs heavy on the city. Wet days in Los Angeles are unusual. They are the days locals grumble about everyone else's inability to operate a motor vehicle. The best days in LA are the days after a rain, when the mountains crisply show their beauty, breaths freshen, moods shift, and people smile. These are the great days, when it's easy to feel invincible and hard to see anything otherwise.

I was twenty-eight years old and working as a delivery driver for a local beverage company, driving an eye-catching, bright blue branded van all around town delivering cases of flavored water to the owner's closest relationships. It was a Friday. On Fridays I had four deliveries. In my company polo and khaki shorts, I loaded seventy cases, flipped the radio to the tune of '90s hip-hop, and pulled out of the storage facility. First turn, cases flew everywhere. I had forgotten to strap them down. Again. I believe that's "shaken, not stirred."

What was great about my job wasn't solely the fact I attracted the ladies in my charmingly colored creepy van, but the fact that I could live a life as an artist and still survive without having to wait another table. Being able to leave the flashers on in a loading zone while going in for an audition is a major plus in this city. And reciting lines while walking through a cubicle-filled office building with an eight-case loaded dolly proved to be an effective (and popular) memorization technique. On this particular Friday, I had one personal stop at the end of my route. Today, the van would be parked on the residential streets of the UCLA campus, just behind the medical center. It was infusion day.

Work clothes to suit to work clothes to gym clothes to work clothes again. The van was my Clark Kent to Superman's phone booth. Except I was in the back of a windowless van, falling over while struggling to get a pant leg around each foot and working up an oxygen-eating sweat. Today was work clothes to comfortable patient wear. In my world, that meant my favorite sweats and a hoodie, the most comfortable combo on this piece of Southern California earth. As the side door slid open and I burst out in a panic for fresh air, a pair of class-destined students screamed and split directions as they ran away in horror. With that, I was on my way to another appointment.

Walking past the campus dorms revived memories of my carefree years at Auburn University. Construction ahead closed the sidewalk, forcing me to cross the street. The sight of a crew pouring concrete gave me a flash of my family, generations of construction men passing in my mind's eye. A few distracted steps later, I came back to reality in front of a closed restaurant. I stopped. Thoughts of my time waiting tables moved through my mind as I looked into the dark, empty space. Focus pulled to my reflection in the front window. It was as if my life was reflecting back to show me this rail-thin, weakening man.

152 pounds

Thoughts of the apparition carried me to the front of the UCLA medical center. As white jackets and blue scrubs passed, so did a forever feeling. Here I was, once again. Back in this place. With a deep breath and a reassuring smile, reality sank in. Not one person, other than the staff, likes hospitals. They are cold and scary places, filled with waiting and uncertainty, sadness and the harshest truths. My reality was that it was time for another treatment.

The door opened into a quietly quick-flowing space filled with a receptionist's desk to the right, a few vacant seats to the left, nurse's stations leading to other rooms along the side, and a line of sectioned-off, divider-separated treatment spaces overlooking a beautifully landscaped courtyard. I was there because of my Crohn's disease, and the treatment was an infusion of Remicade. Treatment three of a scheduled six. In the times prior, the four-recliner section was all mine. "We like to keep patients going through different situations separate, for respect," a nurse once told me. This wasn't a space for just people with Crohn's. Cancer and chemo were the majority. On this particular day it was busier than normal, and while waiting, watching the station being cleaned and prepared, my mind again drifted.

I was in front of the hospital, a month and a half ago. The first infusion. A little over three years to the day after nearly dying, and I was on my way to another medication. Another form of treatment. Still living the same life. Still following the same routine. Still indulging in the same habits. Still living with Crohn's disease. Scared? A little. Uncertain? Fully. I had gone through a lot and put others through a lot, so I had decided not to share with anyone when my infusions would take place. At that very moment, I wished I had. With a deep

6

breath and thoughts of the past pounding, I moved one leg reluctantly in front of the other. Time slowed. The elevator doors closed. The floors rose. The corner turned. The door approached. The knob reached for itself. When suddenly, a voice came from behind.

"Hey! You walked right past me, you dummy!"

She was there. She came anyway. How did she know the day and time? Didn't matter. My heart rose and my face swelled. The love of my life had put her life on hold. "Thank you for coming, babe," I said as she stood there with her endearing smile, my favorite chocolate, a magazine, and a reassuring hug. If she only knew how alive her touch felt that day. How truly grateful I was to have her there.

"You think I was really going to let you do this alone?"

I've never wanted to be a burden to anyone. Unfortunately, too often I was. I've also always held everything in, creating isolation and refusing help. Mad, yet never fully understanding why. But people do show up. Learning to see that, accept it, and let them in was something I had yet to understand. She showed up. For treatment one and for treatment two.

Unfortunately, on this particular Friday, treatment three, her work would not allow that surprise. At the same time, this wasn't the unknown anymore. It wasn't scary and the uncertainty had faded. This was the next phase of my existence. Alone or not.

"Mr. Godsey. We're ready for you."

Over I walked and into the recliner I climbed. Settling in and looking up revealed a woman in her midfifties sitting in the adjacent recliner. She was receiving an infusion as well, chemotherapy. Her second

7

bout of breast cancer. In fact, today was her last treatment. The cancer came back and she had fought it off yet again. With her infectiously inspirational personality, it was obvious why.

The nurse wiped my arm. "Ohhhhh." She perked up as if I just gave her a meltingly suave look. "You have great—"

Here we go again. "I know, I know. I have great veins." An industry-accepted excitement for the nursing community. To that, she started the drip and set the clock.

120 minutes

Two hours of thoughts and confusing outcomes were happily interrupted by a soft voice from that adjacent recliner.

"What are you healing from today?" Her smile invited anxiety's relief and a support for my growing lonely feeling. Our conversation moved into our battles and survivals. Family and work. Our stories and surgeries. We talked strength and faith. Emotions and truth. Food and lifestyle. She was an amazingly honest woman with good values and a deep appreciation for the day she was given. The kind of person you remember.

Through a great conversation's swift passage, her timer rang and the nurse unhooked her. She rolled down her sleeve and that was it. Into forever it would have to be. Her last treatment was over. The lady had beaten cancer twice and was quitting her job. She was finally going to focus on helping others through a nonprofit she had always been a part of but never fully committed to. She was also looking forward to appreciating every day with her grandchildren. Gathering herself, she picked up her sweater, turned back, and looked at me with her bold green eyes of strength.

"You'll find your way through this. Stay willing."

And with that lasting thought, our paths divided.

For that last hour, I sat there and thought about her while consuming the free chips and apple juice. I say 'free' because the hospital so nicely provided them. On some bill, they were probably several thousands of dollars. The flowers were landscaped to perfection, perfectly grown and shaped. Outside of that minor, distracted thought, everything the woman said started to sink in, although most of it wouldn't make sense until years later. I walked into that place, again prepared to tackle it alone, and again, life had put someone there. It does that, when you're available to see it.

"Beep, beep, beep."

Like the horrific sound of a code blue panicking in my ear, the treatment was over. The nurse unhooked me.

"We'll see you in six weeks, sweetie!"

Halleluiah. I made it. Staying strong and following the prescribed path. Now, back to my normal existence as a starving artist. Polos, auditions, and water deliveries. Living to the fullest what any late-twenty-year-old believes life to be. Enough experience to enjoy the days but never really understanding the implications of the life being led. But who does until you've led it?

Over the next couple of days my dream of finally being healthy vanished. My body began to ache and weaken. I developed a rash on

9

the right side of my torso that quickly expanded from the spine to the belly button. By day three, the pain stretched from my right shoulder to my foot. Extremely concerned, I called my doctor's office and scheduled an emergency appointment with the gastroenterologist.

Arriving at the nurse's station and showing them the rash, speculation formed around shingles, a highly contagious disease that immediately made the world back away from exposure. All I cared about was getting medicine to relieve the excruciating pain, not the bubble-boy treatment that was already much too familiar to this battered body. The rash itched severely and hurt with every breath, scratch, and shift of clothing. Shortly after being quarantined, the doctor came in. She examined and confirmed it was a terrible case of shingles.

"I knew you would probably get shingles."

"Wait, what?"

"Shingles are very common with this medicine."

Well, that was news to me. This was the first time shingles had ever been mentioned. The commercials always show the elderly, not a twenty-eight-year-old. I was so confused. How could this happen? Why didn't they tell me this was a possibility? A normal case of shingles, ok, I could maybe handle that. A terrible case of shingles, I'm not happy. A terrible case of shingles on top of everything I had already gone through? Terrified. I felt lied to, deceived.

"I'm going to push back your infusions until this clears up and then we'll continue with the final three."

Wait a second. I have to take medicine to clear up a reaction that the other medicine caused, then go back to the infusion medicine again?

Healing one section of my intestine or not, what was this doing to my body? A million questions filled my mind through every word she spoke from then on. Slowly coming into focus was the realization of why I had chosen to go forward with the treatments in the first place. Slowly, I had been justifying a way to continue on with my lifestyle. Until she spoke the last words I ever remember her saying.

"There's a good chance the shingles will come back in the future. But we need to stay on the medicine. It's the only way for full remission."

That's when it hit me. My past, the lady, the doctors all flashed through my mind. After decades of suffering, it finally became clear. The dots connected. Crohn's disease is an autoimmune disorder. Meaning my immune system had been compromised. If I was taking medicine to control the disease, and the medicine was, in turn, weakening my immune system even further to the point where a disease that normally lies dormant until the twilight years of life, then what comes next? Something I probably can't come back from.

2 months

Two months it took to heal from those shingles. Two months of agony and thoughts about how to finally put control into my own hands.

Me: "How did you do it?"

Her: "Beat cancer twice?"

Me: "Yeah."

Her: "If you want to heal, you have to believe you can, have a great support system and faith in every day from here forward."

Her words echoed, and that was my…

1 last treatment

11

CHAPTER 2: Back to the Beginning

During the summer of 1983, life in the modest midwestern city of Niles, Michigan was beginning for one, and beginning again for two. A daughter, freshly back in the world, joined her parents for a night out. A man, recently reconnected to his roots, embraced his friends for the same. The place would be an old-fashioned street dance, where police barricaded Main Street and local vendors lit the mood with food and flowed the blues with booze. As the rhythm's twists turned, their eyes connected.

A week later, Mark packed a bottle of wine, paired it with a mild cheddar cheese and crackers, rolled up a few blankets, and arrived at Gayle's door just as the clock turned on time. He then drove her to where the high grass met the soft beige sand, and their first date was on a blanket overlooking the setting sun of a majestic Lake Michigan summer night. The cool breeze cuddled them into the blankets as crashing waves relaxed in the fading light's rays. He pulled out the wine. She swooned at the sight of him. He pulled out the cheese. She smiled at his charm. She was completely enthralled.

Just then, she noticed the bottle was already open? He caught her reaction and said, "This is my grandfather's homemade wine." Curiosity drifted her eyes to the cheese, which revealed a missing corner, imprinted with teeth marks. Trying to keep the wheels on, Mark exclaimed in panic, "I didn't eat lunch!" Deflecting, he poured the wine, clinked her glass, nervously took a large gulp of his drink, and said, "This is life."

She smiled, put the glass to her lips, drank, and spit. It was terrible. I mean, come on. Homemade wine from your grandpa shouldn't have the highest standards to begin with. Nevertheless, as they say, love is blind. So blind that a month later, while at a classy steakhouse and between the salad bar offerings of crumbled blue cheese and kidney beans, he got on one knee, pulled out a box, and proposed. Not the least bit surprised by this point, she said yes.

Because love is more than a sour bottle of wine and nibbled block of cheese. Love is a connection to the same trustful feeling, and on an unpredictably warm and sunny November day of that same year, they wed in a quaint countryside church. Making their new beginnings and fresh start official.

A little over a month later, Target was running a sale. Or at least that's what she told her new husband. After all, shopping relieved the extreme nausea she had been experiencing. No, not from the recent wedding. She was actually feeling ill. A few days prior she had visited her doctor and they ran tests. Today she would get the results. She was to call at 2 p.m. So, what's the best way to keep your mind occupied when life has you stressed? For most, detrimental comfort foods. For her, shopping.

Two p.m. rolled around, and she went outside to a glass structure on the sidewalk, put a few coins in the slot of a solid box, grabbed the receiver attached to a metal coil, and pushed ten digits on the number pad. I believe they called these relics "pay phones." The office answered, and the doctor got on the line.

"Mrs. Godsey. Congratulations. You're pregnant."

By late August 1984, the man and wife had done all the classes, she was eating what they presumed was a healthy diet, they were keeping up with the practices of the times, and everything was going according to plan. The pregnancy was very much routine for the era. She had only gained twenty-five pounds and stayed active throughout. Life was perfect.

In the hospital waiting room, both sets of grandparents watched through a tiny window, patiently waiting while looking down the hall. After only an hour of prep, and fifteen minutes of delivery, the nurses cleaned off the baby, administered the standard shots and vaccines of the time, and placed him in the arms of his new mother and father. Mark and Gayle were now proud parents of a beautiful baby boy— me.

Mark ran down the hall, turned the corner to the onlooking grandparents, and with a smile shouted, "Piece of cake!" Unbeknownst to him, that day would be the last piece of cake for their new piece of cake.

CHAPTER 3: Infancy

Two days after settling into a freshly reformed family of five, I started projectile vomiting. The doctor determined it to be an allergy from my dairy-based formula. After various recommendations and personal decisions, a different formula was decided upon. I was shifted from dairy-based formula to soy without hesitation, again dismissing the option of my mother's nutrient-rich, beneficial bacteria–building, natural breast milk. A new life was in the hands of an era's evolving science.

A baby develops in its mother's womb for nearly ten months. It is fed and grows from her nutrients and the assistance of her bacteria. Milk and soy formulas contain manufactured nutrients to replace what an infant would receive through breastfeeding—nourishment taken away from the mother and put into the hands of lab-generated and altered substances. Modified organisms versus naturally occurring genetic elements. This, and the practices of whisking away the baby after birth and washing it when the baby should be left to breathe and live in its mother's essential bacteria, then administering recommended or standard shots and vaccines, played a role in the underdevelopment of my microbiome. I was exposed from the beginning. It didn't necessarily cause what happened next, but it did wear me down into the eventual reveal. One thing at a time, connecting over the course of time.

The solution—the new formula—was the choice of the times, and with it, we could finally be a family. Life happily moved on for the next seven months, until one night when I developed a 104°F fever. This happens to many babies at some point in their infancy and so was nothing to worry about. Until the fever carried through the next day. My parents decided the emergency room was the best option. My first hospital sleepover since birth. A five-night sleepover that was eventually diagnosed as acute bilateral cervical lymphadenitis. The doctors performed a spinal tap to rule out any possibility of spinal meningitis and prescribed my first doses of antibiotics (that I am aware of).

Acute bilateral cervical lymphadenitis is an infection, usually of the upper respiratory tract, and is known as "strep" throat. There are other, more fatal, ailments (like cat scratch disease) that are usually the first ones to be tested for when this type of infection is present. Ruling those out, the vast majority of the rest get the upper respiratory or "strep" diagnosis. After that, it's up to the doctor what to prescribe. Antibiotics are often the first choice, as they were in my case.

Thankfully, it wasn't spinal meningitis or whatever that crazy cat scratch disease is. Couldn't I just be a baby already? I hadn't even smashed my face into the cake of my first birthday yet. I was still bald and pale white. Crying through the night. Depriving my parents of sleep. Typical for any baby. But it was another illness for this one. I was now battling ear infections. Recurrent, severe ear infections. Each episode resulted in a dose of antibiotics or similar medicine, and each time wore my body down more and more. After repeated infections, the doctor decided to insert tubes. I was just two years old.

Ear infections are not uncommon for babies. They often follow a common cold or viral infection. Many people experience ear infections between the ear drum and what is known as the eustachian tube, which connects the ears, nose, and throat, making it easy for a cold to connect and infect throughout the ear.

Let's take a second and connect these dots: rejection of dairy milk led to soy versus my mother's, followed by an upper respiratory infection, and topped off by recurrent ear infections. Connected to the immune system, originating from the gut, and resulting in infections in the ears, nose, and throat. All treated with antibiotics to kill invading and impeding bacteria. Like an atomic bomb, antibiotics eliminate good inhabitants along with the bad. Antibiotic atomic bombs can't dictate who lives or who doesn't. They just drop, dissolve, and explode, wiping clean everything in its path.

All this before the age of two. During the most crucial time of my life, when my body was supposed to be building up all the important bacteria for the rest of my life, it was fighting to run properly. It was a system being set up to fail from the beginning. The birthing practices, ingredients in the formula, soy, antibiotics, environmental toxins, and every medicine used to treat my ailments in the first couple of years, left me exposed for the rest of my life. It could've happened at age eight, fourteen, or twenty-nine, but for me, it started at birth.

CHAPTER 4: Childhood

Adam Smith, the father of "modern" capitalism, once said: "No society can surely be flourishing and happy, of which the far greater part of the members are poor and miserable." He also noted: "Man is an animal that makes bargains: no other animal does this—no dog exchanges bones with another."

Both statements are true and deeply embedded within our culture. Free enterprise creates endless products, products made by companies looking for the most affordable location for manufacturing and looking to maximize their bottom line. It's the same way we all find the places we call home. Apartments, houses, storefronts, high rises, factories, all exist within the confines of a budget. Cities offer breaks and bargains to lure in industry. Industry brings jobs. Jobs bring people. People build families. Families circulate earnings.

Industry brings wealth to a society.

In small towns, community is everything. Your door stays unlocked. Your kids ride bikes in the streets with their friends. Schools bring locals together through academics, sport, and spirit. Work is the day that makes the town alive at night. Community becomes family.

In 1916, a heavy-machinery manufacturer relocated from Chicago to a small southwest Michigan town. They made fork lifts, truck axles, front end loaders, and in the '50s a style of trolley car that would be used in the New York City public transportation system for twenty years. Their name would establish as Clark Equipment.

In 1930, legendary Notre Dame football coach Knute Rockne was suffering from poor health during his last season. As a result, he was losing his voice. No longer able to yell at practice, he sought out two local radio engineers to fix the problem. The engineers needed to design him some sort of PA system. He called it his "electric voice." In the days after his jubilant praise of it, Electro-Voice was incorporated. Since then, they've grown into a renowned electronics manufacturer, maintaining the same values of quality over quantity in the products they established decades prior.

Explorers Lewis and Clark carved a path connecting the east coast to the west. Railroads expanded the paths by decreasing time with increasing power. Interstates and highways put the power into the hands of the people with the cars they operated. The auto industry developed a nation by providing convenience to all. Their product not only made everyday life easier, it also created jobs. Automobiles require parts, parts that would come from as far away as the cheapest contract. As a result, machine shops flourished in midwestern towns, providing the residents with trades and careers for decades. A variety of industry brings a variety of skills and ultimately builds a community into a well-rounded society, one that grows with the families they create.

In the Redbud City of Buchanan, Michigan, Clark Equipment, Electro-Voice, and the machine shops brought light to the city streets for well over half a century, creating a lively town full of traditions, safe neighborhoods, and celebration of achievement. But in the 1980s, the cheapest contracts could be found elsewhere. Promises to labor unions held profits underwater. Communication became computer-based. Business evolved into an easily accessible worldwide economy fueled by growth and sustained by the bottom line. The contracts became outsourced and shipped. Industry shifted to survival, and as a result, companies like the ones in Buchanan found new homes and owners, either overseas or elsewhere, leaving a majority of their employees to do the same. With lost jobs came lost cash flow, and lost cash flow cripples societies. All that remained were empty buildings, unmaintained sidewalks, and dollars turned into dimes. Times like these expose the true heart of a community. Larger cities can absorb the shock by replacing the lost, but smaller communities like Buchanan are forced to find their resilience while avoiding desperation.

As industry was moving out, the Godseys were wheeling in, in their brown Astro van. They turned right on Moccasin Street, traveled less than a mile down a hill, passed a playground and the elementary school, and arrived at their new home, a nearly one hundred-year-old, colonial-style house. This house, ironically, was once owned by Electro-Voice's founder. It was ready for a family of five plus their dog and cat to bring it to life again. The small town of 5,000 people, three stop lights, and hollow spaces was forced to show its grit. The street dances, like the one my parents made first glances at, faded as the noises silenced and planning went to work.

When time shows its fists and throws its punches, connecting a body to the canvas, the true strength is in the hands that lift the body back up and reach out to touch gloves once again. Over the course of the twenty years my family lived in that community, the passion of its citizens happily and repeatedly held the body off the canvas. Money may decide who is rich or who is poor, just as Adam Smith implied, but what Smith failed to understand is a strong community like Buchanan, one that shows faith beyond wealth and compassion beyond doubt. Buchanan, then and now, revealed itself to be a fervent city of hardworking, good, tough, family-oriented people. That was no different for the family my parents were raising and the families that raised them.

It took years to understand how lucky I really was to have the kind of childhood my parents provided. I thought we had the world until I saw what the world had. Now, I realize it was because they worked hard to make the world we had great, and the community kept our world together. I grew up in a family consisting of several generations of entrepreneurs, mainly in some form of construction. My great-grandfather, grandfather, and father owned a family concrete business from 1949 until my dad sold it in 1995. My mom's father, Marvin Selge Sr., started his construction business in 1950. My uncle still successfully runs it today. Luckily, all of my grandparents were friends and golf buddies. Grandpa Selge fought in World War II and earned a bronze star for his bravery during the Battle of the Bulge. My other grandfather, Minor Austin Godsey Jr., was drafted into the Marines during the Korean War. Because of his college degree, athletic skills, and parents' farm discipline past, he was placed in a noncombat role.

Unfortunately, my mother had given birth to two other boys, both older than I and both just as you would expect two brothers to be with regard to the things they did to their younger brother. Our household was actively insane. Or insanely active. There was an age gap of six, ten, and thirty years between the other boys and me, which often meant going to several fields or gyms in a single day. We traveled frequently, spent a lot of time with extended family, and all helped the oldest boy—my dad—in some way with his businesses. My role was climbing on machinery and getting yelled at for being in the way, or looking through the mechanics' naked-women calendars hanging just to the left of the red toolbox.

On the days I went to work with Dad, mainly when I was between four and eight years old, we would leave before the sun even showed a morning stretch. On the way, we'd always stop at the coffee shop. He'd talk to the locals (usually his childhood friends) while I picked out a sprinkled donut, chocolate donut, and a rotation of either a glazed twist, bear claw, or jelly filled. And a carton of chocolate milk, the one with the cleverly marketed rabbit on the front. Some days, we'd get a box filled with a variety of glazed, sprinkled, filled, powdered, and puffed. Those were usually job site days. We'd cruise from job to job with the windows down, singing the good times (for Dad. Classics to me). Days at the plant, apart from the equipment climbing and naked pictures, entailed sneaking my way back to the batch plant, where the trucks were loaded with concrete and the old Coke machine provided free product. Free product I happily drank behind one of the parked trucks. Over the course of my youth, I drank a lot of soft drinks, Cokes, soda (pop, as we northerners call it). Whether it was sneaking to the batch plant, semi-frozen in our garage during winter, riding to the gas station or beyond, soft drinks were a happy part of our lives.

My mom, a selfless woman who was and still is a great cook, loved to cook for us. Smell and taste memories of sibling fights over her apple pancakes outside our wilderness-parked camper stay just as sweet with time's passing. We were on the go so much that we ate out often and often ate easily accessible foods. In the same way every average person or family indulges, we lived through the food and lifestyle available to us. Meat, potatoes, dairy, corn, soda, fast food, processed food, and so on. We learned nutrition. We trusted the standard nutrition. We ate what was marketed to us. Especially cheese. The Godsey family has an infatuation with cheese.

Speaking of healthy eating and family influence on a growing child, my snowbird grandparents were flying home after a winter in Florida. My dad was holding me as we looked out the window by their gate. Their plane was landing and he said, "There they are. Do you see them?" To which I replied no, I couldn't see them anywhere. Joining the conversation from the side was an elderly lady with a cliché craggily old-woman voice: "Well you should eat your carrots! Carrots help you see." The three-year-old young gentleman to whom she was speaking looked at her and replied, "You p---y!" (too vulgar to repeat, but it's another word for a female's most sacred space). My dad, in shock, horror, and in one motion turned to his right, calmly walked away, and screamed my brothers' names.

My brothers taught me several of my first words and bad habits. Like my first phrase: "Puck you." I was easily angered and couldn't yet enunciate "F." Then there was that time they locked me in my parent's bedroom with a bungee cord tied to my opposing bedroom's door handle. Every time I tried to open it, it snapped back. They left me with some pop and my favorite junk food while they threw a party downstairs. My parents were on vacation. They thought their jailing bribes were enough to silence the unsilenceable. Great babysitters they were. Told on them I did. But they didn't get into trouble. I actually think my dad laughed at their ingenuity.

Where were we? The whole airport situation. That's right. Looking back now, maybe that nosy old lady was right; I should've eaten more carrots versus extra-large bowls of cereal and milk. Knowing what I do now and how carrots soothe the stomach and digestive tract while

23

providing essential cell-repairing vitamins, there was some truth to her advice. I bet she never gave it again though.

For the first couple of years in our new home I stayed relatively healthy, until around the age of five when I developed a hard-hitting case of the measles. That was followed at age six by hives and rashes in response to certain foods. For the longest time we thought it was because of canned tuna fish. That was a "guesstimation" my parents made based on one main ingredient of many I had consumed that day. We never truly knew. Later—twenty-two years later—my allergy tests would show no allergy to tuna. I know allergies change as a person changes, but I never felt I was allergic to tuna. But this was how it went back then: We all guessed what it might be, treated the symptoms with medicine, and avoided the supposed culprit. Lesson understood now. It's nobody's fault. Just how you live and learn and learn because you get to live.

It may be obvious by now that I've had a lifelong problem with sweets. Sneaking Cokes, donuts, bribery, boxes of cereal in one sitting, pancakes, and more. Sugar is easily my longest-running downfall in the health show that is my life, so much so that while still in diapers, or in this instance without, I would walk next door with only my boots on to get one piece of butterscotch candy. When it came to sweets, I had no shame. As I got older I worked my way down the street to Mr. and Mrs. Dicks' house. I'd knock on the door and Millie, a kind elderly lady who by that time in her life had gone blind, would answer. She'd invite me into their back room just as John was coming around the corner with a glass bowl of m&m's and a scooper, telling me to "hold your hands out." They loved the visits just as much as I did that scoop.

24

Through school, I was a great student, a model for other students. Valedictorian, 4.0, never missed a day, and member of the most studious clubs. Actually, that's a lie. That was my friend. I was an average student who talked a lot, fooled around even more, and watched the clubs meet as I made my way to the principal's office. Standing on "the wall" for recess was my usual position, and talking my way to some sort of discipline was nothing uncommon. "Paper, rock, scissors, shoot. Ok, I'll take the Godsey kid." These were the games my next year's teachers would play, as I was easily that year's last pick.

My mom didn't pack a lunch for us. Not because she didn't want to. She's the type of person who would go outside in a blizzard to start your car on a frozen winter morning because you were running late. She didn't pack a lunch because it wasn't cool to have a boxed lunch. Nobody worth talking to brought bagged carrots and a ham and cheese on white bread. You had Wednesday's nacho day! Every first Thursday's Rib-b-q! Monday's chicken nuggets! The occasional popcorn shrimp! And so deliciously on and on. As kids, we lived for those foods. The French bread pizza. Or the sausage, egg, and cheese English muffin breakfast sandwiches after 5 a.m. baseball practice. School lunches were not the cause of my health issues, but they were a contributor to my exposure. I never once remember anything fresh, or any sort of balance. Balance was prepackaged foods that fit nicely into the divided areas of a Styrofoam tray and were delivered frozen from the food service company. These were eating habits we learned to be ok. From food we saw only one way. If English teaches you English, then lunch time teaches you lunch time behaviors, both of which build into lifelong routines.

It's safe—and probably an understatement—to say my family was and still is sports-oriented. My Grandpa Godsey was recruited and played one season for the Indiana Hoosiers basketball team, until a knee injury ended his career. My uncle, Marvin Selge Jr., was a standout running back and played in college. My dad enjoyed coaching a number of our teams and was only good at the games that didn't count, like pool, darts, and shuffleboard. Ok, this one time I'll give him credit; he was a great tennis player and one hell of a basketball shot (but, between us). And I spent my elementary school years watching my brothers play football and baseball.

Naturally, by being around it as often as I was, and loving to play, sports were a large part of my childhood, whether it was my grandpa teaching me his outdated one-handed jump shot, yelling at the screen during Indiana games, taking me to the Twins and Red Sox spring training every year, or forcing my dad to shoot baskets for hours and throw one more "grand finale" pop up over and over again. I loved games and was—still am—passionate and competitive playing them. Sometimes a little too competitive. Hey, nobody in their honest mind likes to lose. I'm an imperfect perfectionist. Second, third, or tenth place trophies don't exist.

In 1992, the Indiana Hoosiers were #1 in the nation. It was a Tuesday night in early February. My TV was tuned to channel 11. The Indiana State Farm lady led the program off with her traditional singing of the fight song while sweeping the tunnel of the stadium's floor. "Oh Indiana, my Indiana..." The battle in this game was one like never seen before. It started with the teams repeatedly trading the lead. From Hoosier Court in the House of Godsey I parroted the announcers while playing along to the flow of the game with the

Indiana-branded mini hoop attached to the back of my bedroom door. Despite tightening lungs, Godsey put on a performance for the ages. Dunks from the bed. Passes off the wall. Threes from the window. Down by one point with seconds left in the game and lungs now closing with wheezing pain, I brought the ball down the court for one last shot. I could barely take in another breath but played on. Just as the buzzer was sounding and the defense was hounding, the shot went up and I collapsed.

This time my lungs were closed. The wheezing held the tightness. I grasped for air as we pulled into the hospital's emergency roundabout. Three heavy doses of albuterol later, I jittered free. Jittery from the steroids. Free from the grip of dying to inhale air. I was ten years old. A later follow-up with a specialist diagnosed it as "sports-induced asthma." Over the course of twenty years I was prescribed an assortment of inhalers, disks, steroids, albuterol, prednisone, and so on and so abused. I used an assortment of them religiously. Attacks came so often that my dad found it cheaper to buy a machine that administered the albuterol versus constantly paying more and spending countless hours in the emergency room. I lived off this machine. It was another safety blanket until I was in my late twenties. Two decades on that machine, those inhalers, the disks and steroids or prednisone, all to calm the lung inflammation. Have you ever watched a fish labor to breathe when it's out of the water? That's asthma. Oftentimes mixed with the feeling of someone stepping on your chest.

Asthma is generally attributed to seasonal allergies, and prednisone is a commonly used tool to calm various forms of inflammation in the body. Side effects of most medicines used to treat asthma frequently contribute to anxiety and mood disorders. In this second decade of the twenty-first century, over 15 percent of the population in the United States suffers from some form of asthma. That's a lot of reactions to pollen and seasonal allergies. Through living with the sometimes embarrassing and far too frequent struggle of asthma, and the knowledge I've gained after cleaning out the toxins from my lifestyle and diet, I disagree with "sports induced" and partly agree with "seasonal allergy." Asthma is inflammation created from the body trying to cope with the chaos caused by the toxins we breathe. Asthma is also associated with infection and the closing of airways due to an imbalance in the immune and digestive systems. Activities and changes of season trigger an already vulnerable system. Everything we breathe and eat that's made of toxic substances ultimately affects our lungs because the toxic substances wear down the immune system and expose the body in some way. This is also known as our "toxic load."

Here's another thought: If my asthma was sports induced, then how come I was hospitalized on so many occasions from exposure to cats? Or a live Christmas tree? Or certain candles or smells or foods? Or toxins? Like the time I bleached my hair blond to show team unity for our soccer state tournament and nearly died from the fumes. Dad still shakes his head at that one.

These are the growing pains of growing up, right? Sickness finds us all, and as the body develops, pains come and go. It's just a normal part of life. Between the ages of twelve and sixteen, young males grow faster than at any other time of their life. I was over six feet tall by the age of sixteen. The pain in my hips was constantly uncomfortable. It got to the point where…well this is obvious: I went to the doctor. He examined me and determined that one leg was longer than the other and that I should put a lift in my shoe. Lift I did, and pain it stayed. The lift found its way out after a few months and the pain finally found its way out a couple of years ago. Around the age of thirty.

How about another growing pain of growing up? A child's third-worst nightmare outside of the doctor and that thing in the closet at night. The dentist. I hated the dentist! Cavities and teeth issues have been an ongoing problem. After all, I did eat a lot of sugar. And sugar is the main cause, right? There wasn't a time I could remember going to the dentist and not having some form of cavity or breaking down of a tooth. It was embarrassing, feeling like I was a failure because of my teeth. In actuality, my dentist loved me; he thrived from my situation. When I was sixteen, I needed a root canal for an abscess in my mouth. I was put on antibiotics to treat the infection (again) and received my first crown.

The connection between my mouth and my immune system issues didn't begin to become apparent until after I was diagnosed with Crohn's disease. That same childhood dentist made a comment about how his patients with digestive issues—like IBS, colitis, and Crohn's— all had similar dental issues and patterns. I only fully grasped the connection when I was formulating the changes to healing. Digestion starts in the mouth. Bacteria builds from there and affects everything.

Through high school, my ailments increasingly worsened. At that point, I had a mouth full of lead and a pocket full of asthma, and every fall I came down with some form of serious infection or immune system issue such as sinus infections, hives, ulcers, or worse. One fall, while in the middle of a drill at soccer practice, I suffered severe

29

pin-pricking cramping in my abdomen. I left practice and, per our routine, Dad and I found our way to the hospital. By this time, I should've had my own private wing: "The Godsey Suite, a living and breathing medical mystery." Over the course of the standard treatment for the immediate symptoms came the prognosis and explanation. I was now suffering from what the doctor believed to be an overgrowth of yeast in my intestines. An overactive fungus. The prescription was antibiotics. Again.

Outside of the overactive yeast issue, the hives that had been slowly starting to present themselves in my earlier years then took over. My entire torso and arms became covered with them. Again, off to the family practitioner we went. He administered a shot of cortisone, wrote a prescription for an antibiotic (again), and sent us on our way. I stood up from my wheelchair to say goodbye to the receptionist, and the whole world went dark. That was my first experience blacking out. The strength of the shot was too much to leave so soon.

The cortisone ending up helping. The hives healed, and to celebrate, my favorite meal! Mom's mastacholi. Noodles, pasta sauce, cheese, cheese, and more cheese. Baked to perfection. Served on a large plate and consumed, three sittings' worth in one. After all, we were "growing boys." Appetites in our (nearly) all-boy household were large and grocery receipts were long. Through it all I remained rather thin (usually around 170 pounds) due to being active, or so I thought.

Over the course of that month a terrible pain grew in my throat and chest. I could barely swallow the softest of foods or water. As you might imagine, my symptoms and complaining were wearing thin with others. It's hard to express the severity of an illness when you're sick so often. Others would frequently make comments like, "You're too

30

sensitive" or "He's my sensitive friend," phrases I've heard far too many times. But this pain felt like someone stabbing my chest with a jagged sword on every breath. For a couple of weeks the pain remained constant and nobody would believe me.

"Dad, I can't even swallow water it hurts so bad."

"You're overreacting."

I finally convinced someone I needed to go to the hospital, where the doctors decided to do an endoscopy. The result?

"Brandon is suffering from ulcers on his esophagus. I believe this is from herpetic esophagitis." The doctor, unaware of the weeks of pain and complaining and disbelief that led to this point, then stated, "This is a very painful ailment and should be treated with extra caution." Finally, someone understood.

Herpetic esophagitis is a condition where ulcers form on the esophagus, mainly in people who suffer from cold sores or the HSV-1. I had not been diagnosed with HSV-1 and was yet to be sexually active. Kissing I had done plenty of since the second grade, and cold sores that I had subtly developed around the age of fourteen became more prevalent the more my condition worsened, but having an ulcer-filled esophagus was an easy diagnosis, although a blatant error to not examine further. Herpetic esophagitis develops in those who have such a weak immune system it allows the virus—one that's in the same family as chicken pox and shingles—to thrive in your esophagus. Strong immune systems, even if the HSV-1 virus is present, don't suffer from this condition. Regardless, antibiotics, prednisone, and the usual suspects were back and, once again, they healed the immediate and obvious situation. Esophagitis caused by

31

herpes was the doctor's final answer for a virgin with a history of illness and immune-system failures.

The experience taught me that it was up to me to make sure I was being heard correctly. We each walk a unique path, and expecting anyone else to fully comprehend what you've gone through, or are going through, is impossible. We can only half-understand from our own experiences, an outsider's knowledge, and make judgments from there.

That was the fall of the new century, 2000.

As winter rolled around, so did the farmer's almanac prediction, garnering the greatest days for any kid in the north—multiple snow days. One winter, after a blizzard that brought nearly two feet of fresh powder, our Christmas break was extended by two weeks. Seizing every second, my friends and I spent the day plowing paths, building forts, packing snowballs, and strategically placing items around our one-acre, tree-filled, house-in-the-center, lot. As night fell and the moon illuminated the snow, the neighborhood gathered, discussed the rules to the game, and divided.

For hours we dodged, dipped, ducked, and dove our way around that yard. From youngest classmate to oldest brother and his dog biting our ankles, the outside world didn't exist beyond the battle. One of my greatest childhood memories. The game carried on until well after 2 a.m., after which the ones who remained called truce, went inside to find heat, and were greeted by the smell of steamy hot, freshly pulled out of the oven pizza. It's not delivery, it's…the kind of frozen pizza you salivate for, with the thick crust, melting cheese, and hearty ingredients. Hot and ready to be consumed. Just what our exhausted bodies needed. The love and thoughtfulness that only a mother offers at 2 a.m. Never replaced. Never replicated. Never underappreciated. Forever making youthful memories better.

We laughed, ate, warmed up, and talked about the snowball fight for hours. It was the kind of night that keeps the conversation going well into the morning's pajamas, fire, video games, and apple pancakes. That was our house growing up. Three generations of boys. Memories like these keep us humble in our ways, for the rest of our days. The kind of times that take years to fully appreciate their wealth.

Was I sick my entire youth? No. What I was, was living through my ailments. Like we all too often do. Did this affect how I would get to play or live as a youth? Yes. Throwing snowballs while puffing on my inhaler and taking a "bathroom" break was dismissed, ignored in the fun madness of being a kid. Live with what life gives you is our justification for blindly ignoring our aches and pains. Instead we attribute the aches and pains to isolated incidents and treat them that way. Healing from the mindset of getting back to the game as soon as possible. Living while ignoring, rather than treating from exploring. Constantly being sick is a burden, and finding places to keep your mind away from it becomes the goal.

In the spring, my body sprang a leak. It was the last couple months of high school, the end of an illustrious sports career, and the next stage of my health journey. Despite all of my debilitating issues, I was rather decent at sports. I still hold the school record for most errors in a career with our baseball program. I often leave out the part of playing the most games in a career. It's far more fun to make humor of the situation. Despite that, I was fortunate to enjoy soccer, basketball, and baseball enough to excel to a higher level than most.

Spending the majority of my childhood running on the stomachs of my brother's football team, yelling "sexy women in football" as my dad led the workouts, or retrieving foul balls for a piece of gum and playing "run down" or "pickle" behind the dugout of my brother's baseball games, had its benefits. Often, I found myself playing on teams or around kids several years older than I was. This, like anything else, proved beneficial and had drawbacks. Beneficial because it allowed me to develop at a much younger age, and detrimental because of the lasting psychological effects from being around much older minds that were more established than mine. Behind it all, I'm a competitor who loves being a part of a team and loves to play.

FIRST LOVE, FIRST BLOOD

Whether you were fifteen and drawing on your notebook in math class, or twenty-two and walking to the door of a college sorority house for a blind date, or twenty-five and sipping peppermint tea at a coffee shop, wherever you were, whatever you were doing, it met you with the happiest anxiety-filled confusion you'll never experience again, and more than likely, it left you with dry eye sockets and cotton soaked in tears just as fast as it feverishly moved in. We're not ready when it shows its face for the very first time. We don't find it. It finds us when we least expect it. The time you were able to spend in it, whether it stayed or left long ago, replays, rethinks, and relives its way into our memories. Positive times, positive remembrances, positive affection.

First love is never our best love. We're too young to understand its power and too inexperienced to understand ourselves. We're connected in the most uniquely special way life has to offer and disconnected by life having too much to offer. With love comes timing.

34

Timing brings love to crossroads. Paths that divide. Decisions of how to remain, whether to remain. However it comes to us, that very first time, it hits with knee-buckling force and inhaler-taking puffs.

It was a beautiful spring Michigan evening. The sun faded in the blue of fresh air and green of new life. A light dew was settling on the grass. Cleats, chants, bats, and leather gloves captured the sounds of high school baseball. We were in the fourth inning of a Tuesday night game, down by a score of 4–2, and my teammate was at the concession stands scoring hot dogs and after-game dates. "Don't look now but sitting in our stands, over my left shoulder, are three girls from another school who are interested in meeting after the game." I glanced, then he and I connected eyes again; he raised his brow, gave a look and slight nod of accomplishment. "In fact, the blonde one is interested in meeting you. So, don't mess this at bat up, buddy! What's the score?"

In his ever-so-slick suaveness he picked McDonalds as our postgame meeting place. During the teenage navigation of life, McDonalds holds the same value as the place serving the juiciest cuts of filet. The dollar menu would suffice, just as long as the girls are there. In the adult version of life, we justify going or staying while thinking about our comfortable sweats and the binge watching we need to catch up on. Always go. Always, always go. Life shows us only so many doors, and you can't open them by staying in the same room with your chocolate-covered candy popcorn mix and pinot grigio wine. I mean, I don't drink pinot grigio. Anymore.

Walking in stopped time to a moment of beautiful innocence, and there sat that blonde-haired, blue-eyed girl. Neither of us could say much to the other. We didn't understand what was happening. We just understood it was. Possibly because of my teenage gentlemanly habits of eating two double cheeseburgers and a large order of chicken nuggets, washed down with a super-sized Coke. Or possibly because of my conversation-stopping, painfully unfunny teenage jokes delivered at the most inopportune moments? Nervous, I was held by the grip of her beauty and laugh. Eventually we spoke to one another. It wasn't much. It was enough, and that was the beginning of the period of life that was us. First love.

That next morning, my stool changed. The water was no longer clear. There were undigested French fries and lettuce. There was blood. There was I, terrified. I kept it to myself for a couple of days, then eventually brought it up to my friend Mr. Hot Dog during practice, which immediately prompted: "Coach, what would cause blood in your stool? You know, asking for a friend." The conclusion of that conversation led to a diagnosis of the most common scenario, a hemorrhoid flare-up. For the next several years, that's what I thought every time blood colored the water. I had no idea it was actually a step in the process of what was developing in my body.

Measles, rashes, hives, asthma, sinus infections, mismatched legs, abscesses, ulcers, fungus, yeast, bloody stools, and every other common cold and flu, bumps, and broken bones, most of which were treated with some kind of immune system–diminishing medicine or antibiotic. It was wearing me down on the inside while slowly working its way to the outside. Looking back, it's easy to see. My body started off weak and was fed by foods that exposed it even more and treated with medicines that solved the immediate while worsening the overall. A system set up to fail from the beginning.

By the end of high school, I was starting to hear things like, "Man, you have a lot of issues" or "Are you ever healthy?" and "Why is Brandon always so angry?" Comments like that plagued my mind for the next decade. Comments that added up and weighed heavier as they rolled in more often. Had anyone else in my family experienced these issues to this extent? Not really. My grandparents suffered from different forms of cancer later in life, due to tobacco and stress. My dad has had "childhood" asthma, bladder cancer, and heart issues that I fully attribute to his eating, smoking, and lifestyle. My middle brother suffers from asthma. My older brother has remained healthy. My mother has stayed healthy other than heart issues attributed to diet and stress. Nobody though, had the exposure or progression that I did. This is important to understand. Life isn't fair at times. It seems easy to see now what happened over the course of those eighteen years, but eighteen years is a long period of time and the dots were hard to connect. Nearly impossible, especially when living in a society that uses tunnel vision as a reaction to ailments versus acting to find root causes before, or even after, they develop into worse conditions. A society that treats a current illness versus understanding the environment, stress, lifestyle, and medical history. Going through all of that and figuring out what I have, sucks. I suffered a lot, and if things had been different I wouldn't have had to, or at least not suffered as much. I didn't have a voice or a choice then. I just was.

Despite it all, masking the increasing pain while stressing about choices that were already well in motion, blurred the summer heat that was us. What, did you think I was going to just let the love story end like that? Well, in a way, I kind of did.

37

That spring carried through late summer, and in a time when the rest of time moved forward, we lived in the pause of fresh experience. Her innocence and free-spirited soul made anything beyond the present day seem unimaginable, nonexistent. Time was on our side. Wrapped in a blanket on the shores of another pristine Lake Michigan sunset, in a conversation full of youthful desire and imagination. Talking of the future as if it were already here, and our favorites that feel like they've matched us together forever. Anyone who has ever had the experience of first love remembers this. Insignificant conversations transitioning through connected pauses. Kisses that withstand the disconnect of time and space. Feelings that never lose the touch of that embrace. Despite how every moment from then on evolves, this was the only moment to be in.

Life moves so fast that far too often we never grasp the reality of what is right in front of us until years have relegated it to history. The one constant to our existence is that it moves forward. We go, grow, and find it elsewhere, and just as it continuously gives, it selfishly takes away. Life gave us that first love and timing took it away. Decisions had already been made, and at the end of that summer, I left for college a thousand miles away. I left those blue eyes in the summer mist of a memory.

CHAPTER 5: College

In the south, there's a pride in Southern hospitality. Life does move a little bit slower, and conversations unfold under the leaves of oak and magnolia. On the plains sit communities bound together by spirit and faith. The unfortunate past that still lingers in the ideals of a few oftentimes casts a shadow over the heart that exists throughout. The core of the South is a generous and grateful place. Football is the obsession and fall Saturdays spent around family is the devotion. Having a family, people who truly care about you, your time with them and vice versa, traditional or not, is their strength and contentment. Southern hospitality is a family.

College is when we find ourselves finding ourselves for the very first time. On our own. The decisions, what we make of it, and how we live it is in our hands. Cares? Zero. Time is spent learning through the day and cramming everything in at night. College is an exploration within yourself and development through curriculum and socializing. It's a confusing, exhilarating, and intoxicating journey. Reckless habits form and settle in; routines develop from the laziness of not caring to comprehend. Too young to understand and too free to see. The time can make you and easily break you if you're not conscious of it. Don't get me wrong, it's an amazing period. A needed change, an adjustment, and a fresh experience that makes growing old seem impossible.

I believe life revolves around adjusting, timing, and the ability to accept change. You find the right timing when you put yourself in the right spaces for it to find you. In the fall of 2003, I arrived at "the loveliest village on the plains," Auburn University. It was two weeks before classes were to start, but understanding the Auburn culture began four years prior, upon my brother's enrollment. Through action and timing, he gained a job in the football team's video department. After four seasons he graduated and, luckily, was able to line me up to fill his vacancy a semester later. It immediately made my college experience unlike most others.

Early enrollment into the dorms, or at least my dorm, was only for student athletes and staff or girls rushing for acceptance into a sorority. I realized this shortly after my parents picked me up from a morning two-a-day practice and we stood in the registration line outside Mary Lane Hall. I was the only male student in line and clearly remember my dad giving me a subtle look, answered with my smirk. My mom, oblivious, asked, "Do you think you'll like it?" Without hesitation, my dad replied, "I think he'll be ok." This was a three-floor coed dorm and the top two were for the women. I was eighteen; that day felt like heaven. I think I had another blackout. Not that I even knew how to talk to any of them. Confident I played, shy I was. Moved in I did.

Student housing didn't offer much in the way of a kitchen. Small fridges and microwaves found their space in every room. With that, came boxed and easily microwavable foods. Nothing real or fresh. Who has time for that in college? Heat up the ramen, I have a test to cram for. Speaking of tests and studying, my roommate was a laid-back Texan and a highly motivated individual. He spent his time and money prudently during his first year. Classes he often missed, his guitar playing swooned the ladies, and he fought his way through colds and flu. Mid-semester his mom gave him money for a flu shot. He wisely spent it on a case of Corona. He was so happy that night and sick for the rest of the semester. Needless to say, his enrollment lasted one year.

The college environment isn't the most favorable for promoting a strong immune system. After all, this is where people learn all about hangover diets. Greasy food, fried rice dishes, pizza, anything that is quick, cheap, and will "absorb the alcohol." Understanding the effects of alcohol (apart from the fun of inebriation and the horrors of hangover) are unrealistic during this time of life, but alcohol causes inflammation in the body and inflammation ultimately weakens the immune system. Low-quality foods have the same effect. Combined, it's a slippery slope. Flu shots are needed because we live bacteria-depleting lifestyles. It's easier to take the preventative shot than to make the changes needed to strengthen the immune system. Try explaining that to any eighteen-year-old college student.

Auburn is a beautiful campus in a city filled with great people, food, family, football, and traditions. We chant as an eagle circles the stadium before kickoff and roll our famous oak trees at Toomer's Corner after victories. Strange traditions to the outside world, family traditions within. It helped that we had great teams while I was there, and never lost to Alabama, our most hated rival. My job not only allowed me to be directly involved in the football infatuation, it also officially opened the door to explore and develop my skills as a videographer, editor, and content creator. We filmed practices and games, broke down each play for the coaches and players, traveled with the team, and I made highlight films for them to watch after every win. Which were many. Especially against Alabama.

The food in the south is exquisitely enjoyable. Chain restaurants surrounded the college town staples, making access to anything desired seem endless. I would give anything for some of that juicy barbecue right now. There may not be anything in it that fits into my current-day understanding and methods, but despite that, I'll never forget the taste of diced pork smothered with hickory barbecue sauce over two slices of toast and topped with homemade slaw and curly fries. Or the steamed beef and cheese sandwich with a side of pepper Jack–covered Doritos from the hole-in-the-wall place just across the street from the business building. And that fountain Coke. Pop to the old Yankee. Soda to the new southerner.

Eating habits from youth carry into the first time of living on your own. You know, those school lunches in the Styrofoam slots and times spent grabbing "super-sized" combo meals with friends. Without Mom's cooking, this was all I knew. It took years to recognize and deprogram those delicious routines from my everyday habits. Why do we put ourselves through that pain, for just a few seconds of pleasure? Especially when healthy isn't much more of an effort and provides the same satisfaction? Understanding the consequences of the life you've lived is a key factor for seeing the changes and being available to them. Available? I was not. Grasping the monster that was living and growing inside me? I was not.

Fall turned to winter and school took center stage. My days, and commitments, were now having to be planned around the possibility of a sudden and urgent bathroom rush. Over-the-counter solutions masked the root causes. I was taking Tylenol or oxycodone for the pain; my inhaler, the albuterol machine, and disks for the asthma; Mucinex, Benadryl, and nasal sprays for my allergies; and any other prescription that came up to fight off invading infections. And I was

42

drinking more often to cover the pain and confusion that now controlled me.

By the end of the school year my body started to wear down in other ways. Studying became increasingly difficult, and I was now not only having watery, undigested, and oftentimes bloody stools, I was wearing down mentally as well. My brain and body had been deprived of what it needed for so long that the effects of the deprivation were finally building into far worse situations. One concept that is hard to understand while you are in the middle of it is that most health issues take years to develop. We live in a results world, and comprehension of culmination over time is often impossible when immediate relief is so readily available. Like we all do, until faced with a "must change," the destruction train keeps rollin' forward.

In the years following, the sickness extended itself into academic life support. I was no longer required to jam into a half-a-person dorm room, and student on campus housing went to student just off, and apartment living. From mini-fridge to full refrigerator with a sink and dishwasher to match. Not like that was going to change my habits. When we don't have a clue what a "healthy" habit is, it's a little hard to incorporate it into our everyday life, sick or not. Wings, burritos, delivery, drink specials, and leftovers. Work called for many pizza nights in the office. And studying colored the remaining sliver of the pie chart. Life was an unstructured structured routine.

A DAY BEFORE DIAGNOSIS

The alarm clock screamed like a garbage truck backing into a slumbering eardrum. In one disgusted motion, a hand slapped the snooze button—for the third time. Absences and good grades versus sleep and a pounding head. The thought of World History was history and the hangover won again. Sleep would be had until next class at 10 a.m.

By the time the second alarm sounded at 9:30, the gardeners had moved far down the street. Unfortunately, the truck backing into the dehydrated brain carried on its loud pulsating. This time, the lifeless body peeled itself off that bed like a tightly glued sticker to a glass jar. Feeling extreme nausea, and stumbling to the kitchen in search of water, like one magnet to another, my pinky toe so conveniently connected with the edge of the couch. As the saying goes, solve one pain by creating another, a common logic created by someone who obviously never experienced the throbbing of head to toe, literally.

Water poured straight from pitcher to mouth, and like a dying camel finding an oasis, desperation dripped down the front of that deep V-neck. Drifting eyes connected with a pizza box on the counter. With no recollection of whose it was or when it made its way there, it was opened to the euphoric reveal of two slices. Sausage, pepperoni, mushroom, and extra cheese. Still no recollection. Just a laugh at the thought of what was. An alcohol-induced blackout in full effect. My life's newest version of blackouts.

The forceful pounding into every sinus cavity surrounding the brain now mixed with an unpleasant nauseated spinning. The bathroom medicine cabinet held all cures. Last night's irresponsibility was

44

bandaged by four Tylenol washed down with sixteen ounces of mildly warm, fluoride-rich tap water. "I'm never drinking again." Says. Everyone. Ever.

Just then, an agonizingly sharp squeezing took over the abdomen and extended through the bowels. A squeeze that had all too frequently become a sign for system failure. After a ten-minute nap from the spinning, the eyes opened to a body draped over the commode. Glancing while flushing revealed another crimson stool diluted in yellow muck. Hurt and defeat dragged back to the bedroom, and just as the clock changed from 9:59 to 10:00, pain again collapsed to the bed.

On a day like that, a more realistic start time was 11:30, followed by a morning stretch of happiness joyfully extending with the feeling of being able to move. Water, food, and Tylenol, capped off with more sleep, pushed progress for recovery. Showering with Strawberry Morning Mist all-in-one gel washed unknown sins away, and leaving the apartment at 11:47 was right on time for Macroeconomics. Finally pulled together. Sort of.

Exercise at that time was never more than a mile walk at a time. What was once a conditioned athlete running several miles each day turned into a winded, wheezing indolence that could only manage twelve-ounce curls of the cheapest beer possible. Days like today, where two feet dragged the weight of a lifeless torso, were routine. A few blocks, a couple flights of stairs, a few hundred classmates, and one me in the back corner for macroeconomics fate. Just then, the teacher joyfully screamed out, "Test day!"

No way. How could I have forgotten? Again.

The mind wandered into the possibilities of pulling this off. Cheaters never prosper; I was going to fail. My only chance of survival was sneaking out of the fight and, in an unfortunate moment of savior, my stomach hit peak displeasure. The struggling state of wellbeing collapsed into the burning itch of the bathroom routine. Without being noticed, I rushed out of that classroom with the same intensity of what was flushing my system clean.

The hangovers were growing in time, with time, and requiring increasing consumption of Tylenol, Pepto-Bismol, and greasy foods. Thoughts of school again found the rear view to the chicken fried rice of yesterday, trumped by the steak burrito of the day before, and today's treasure of a breaded chicken sandwich, waffle fries, and twelve-pack of chicken nuggets with a side of honey mustard and barbecue sauce. All topped with sixty-four ounces of gut-eating fountain soda.

On this day, the food and medicine calmed my panic and brought into perspective my current predicament's solution. I veered left and headed to the library. "How to finally turn this ship around? This time I'm going to do it. I know I said that last time I would. But this time, I'm for real." You know, those kinds of inspired times that follow hitting reality's pavement.

First off, precious moments that should've been spent studying specific course material were spent in panicked survival mode. Where am I, what do I have, and what is it going to take to get what I need? All while not extending any further than the minimum required. That was the thought process. More time and focus on being prepared wouldn't have allowed that nervous anxiety to justify its invite to an already painful party.

Second, all the time spent plotting the next course of action left only half the time available to spend on tomorrow's requirements. With a body operating this inefficiently, my ability to focus was clouded by intense bouts of mental fog. An ailment that began a decade prior.

"Dad, why does my brain not feel present at times? I feel like I'm here but just physically. A hazy dull reality."

"I suffer this too. Sinuses? Other than that, I really don't know what to tell you."

At this point of college, the dismissed ailment finally grew its name and established: mental fog. Treated with the many-times-rebranded drug known as Adderall. An amphetamine. Three hours' worth of normal studying peacefully understood in one. Adderall, the number one drug not known as a drug and the go-to for anyone needing that extra focus. In my case it was used—not often, not abused, but used, helping me achieve the minimum required for the next day. A bad habit's comfortable reality that expanded in justified uses over time.

Walking the campus, lost in thoughts, a crack in the sidewalk grabbed my foot and I tumbled to the ground. An elbow's collision with the grass gracefully rolled a freefalling body and the inertia of the backpack's swinging sprung it back up as if nothing ever happened. Too late. A sweet and soft Southern voice came to my aid: "Bless your heart! Are you ok?" My campus crush. One of those people you had a class with or would see at the coffee shop periodically and connect with but never seize the signs she was leaving, because you were too lost in yourself. In this case, she was a dorm crush.

"Brandon!" Laughing. "I should've known that was you!"

My face was now as red as the bricks that held the uniform campus buildings in place.

Sincerely, she asked, "How are you?"

"I'm good. My ego's a bit crushed but—"

"It's been forever. Are you doing ok?"

Putting a charm back on the situation: "Yeah, I'm good." Brushing off the leaves and pointing back to the scene of the accident: "That crack jumped out at me!"

Amused but not fooled: "Yeah, sure it did. I haven't seen you since you were sick and took that ambulance to the hospital. I didn't see, but I heard what happened. How are you doing?"

The embarrassment of the sidewalk's crashing froze into the scrambling of not revealing my inner shame of a situation that had faded with time but was still cemented in mind. "Yeah. Thankfully, I got better. My body wasn't doing well." I lied in that moment. I wasn't better and she knew it. An awkward pause ensued.

"Well, we were worried about you. I was worried about you. Anyways, sweetie, I have to get to class. I'm happy to see you're ok, other than that crack. We should get lunch sometime?"

"We should!" Still embarrassed and again missing the opportunity. That was the last time I saw her. Left in the memory of "what if" forever.

My next moment of looking up revealed a six-foot-six, 340-pound lineman leaving the football complex for pre-practice workouts. A future NFL draft pick and intimidating shock to say the least. At the sight of him, my depressing life could be forgotten for a little while. The best parts of the day were taking the pain away. Revived with thirty-two ounces of a blueberry blast sports energy drink and up the spiral staircase I went to the video department's office. Like a child wanting a lollipop in a candy store, my condition screamed for a pit stop and the third stool movement of the day.

As a saying might go, "there's nothing better than a fun and encouraging work environment with a bunch of idiots you love. There's also nothing worse than a toxic one." The substance is in the relationships that form to achieve the job's goals, all while enjoying the company. Walking into the office of the Auburn Video Department was like coming home. There were six student videographers and our boss. Before moving to Auburn, I knew one person whom I had met briefly. That was my boss. My nearest family was five hours away. The others developed into groomsmen and lifelong friendships. Growth happens from stepping outside of your comfort zone and being available to see the beauty that surrounds you while learning through the steps you've already taken. Learned from this day, adapted into present day.

Jokes were commonplace in our office. The radio was our comedy central until professionalism cut the cord. Practice was our getaway, while getting paid. The work may have been extensive, but the relationships and immaturity created a family.

We'd walk to the fields, equipment over shoulder, up the slightly unsettling 40-foot scissor lift, and set up for another night of working to achieve a common goal. A look at the practice script revealed my responsibilities of capturing wide receiver drills, defensive pass rush, and team period.

49

As helmets and shoulder pads crunched, the clock's buzzer rang, signaling the end of pass rush and the beginning of the next period, and my break. As the teams shifted to the other fields, my thirty minutes of freedom shifted to sitting, legs dangling and absorbed in the fading beauty of a fall Southern sky. Enjoyed with a pack of peanut butter cups and that blueberry blast. My phone then flipped open (the "relic" after the relic of those glass "pay phone" things), hit three, send, and called my grandparents. My greatest inspirations. We talked about their winter in Florida, my health, my visit for spring break. She asked about my grades. The only time I would lie to my grandmother. Eventually, "Let me get Grandpa" would be followed by a loud and increasingly annoyed scream of his name: "Austin!" From working around trucks and machinery his whole life and not taking responsibility for the worsening condition, he had lost the majority of his hearing several decades prior. "Hold on, Brandon." The screaming found distance. "Pick. Up. The. Phone." Finally picking up revealing how close she was to his ear before he finally heard her.

"Hello!" A loud and joyful embrace joined the line.

"Grandpa!"

"Hello? Hello?"

We didn't cover much on the phone during those days. It was a family joke for us, but an unfortunate result of stubbornness for him. Whatever the conditions were, I enjoyed hearing their voices and called them nearly every day. Conversations that would sometimes last hours. I never once fully grasped that one day they would no longer exist.

Speaking of something I wished would one day no longer exist, the rushing urgency of my disease instantaneously sprang like the beat of bongos in a subway tunnel. On a day like today, trapped forty feet high with an hour to go, the only answer is cheek squeezing, mind distracting, and keeping the agonizing rush-like contractions in check through paced breathing. I would survive. Unfortunately, from then on, this became me. Became my life.

The beautiful thing about a college town is being able to easily walk everywhere. Or to exercise the practice of "cancel walking." You know, those walks to the frozen yogurt shop because it's healthier than dairy (false) and the exercise allows the reward. Those walks. Except this one was to a cozy bar on the corner of the biggest cross streets of campus—Toomer's Corner. The kind of place you grab a couple tables on the patio and settle in with a group of people you enjoy. The times you feel the most like yourself. The times you are freest to be you. Those spaces of life make you feel good through all spaces of life.

On the street side wall of that patio, my coworkers, their girlfriends, roommates, and I consumed our bonds and laughed our drinks away. "Pass the special, special. Cheers!" Singing "Sweet Home Alabama" unapologetically at the top of our lungs with our glasses in the air and teriyaki, honey barbecue, Jamaican style, Caribbean jerk wings, curly fries, and endless .25 pitchers on the table. Pints clinked and celebrations rang. The best places in life, filled with great-tasting inexpensive food and washed down by chuggingly tolerable inexpensive beer. A perfect combination for any college student.

In a period where you should be fully embracing the moment with your closest, and when all a young adult male can think of is the

51

night's party and the hope for a one-night companion, being distracted by a "sensitive stomach" is a taxing block. By my twelfth wing and I forgot how many beers, the brew factory churned its calling in the gut. This was now the fifth shift change of the day, and it was happening while I was talking to an attractive late arrival who was surprisingly laughing at one of my jokes. At least, that's how it seemed to me. I'm sure to the sober soul it was probably an awkward punchline followed by a random topic for distraction. Doesn't matter. The truth is in the gut and the gut was loudly shouting for attention. I had to get to the bathroom. NOW! So, I politely excused myself and frantically moved through the crowd. Stall time passed, she left, and another moment was lost to the sad truth of the unhealthy reality.

Now with my roommate and college mascot (not in costume). The focus shifted to joining three women while dancing to a locally known band stuck in the tunes of the '80s and cleverly named the Velcro Pygmies. As we pulled into the overfilled parking lot of The Supper Club, my roommate exclaimed, "Those girls are on the dance team!" Winking at me through the rearview mirror, he said, "So, bring your bests, boys! Brandon, have a mint. No offense, but your breath is kickin'! Take one. Take often. Here, take them all!" He always had my back. When I wasn't sick with a cold, I was fighting bad breath and body odor or scratching an overused and irritated crack of my earth region. Again, masking the churning issues with the best-tasting relief. Mints, gum, sprays, and whatever flavor of the week that promised immediate solutions were my embarrassment's saviors.

Upon arrival, and just as any logical person does when they get to the bar before meeting up with people more attractive than they, we ordered shots, raised with one of those clever rhymes that justify the purpose and toasted a "solute." No worries in sight.

"No way these are the girls," I said aloud as three beautiful women walked into the bar. Doubt's justifications started to take over: She's a dancer. I'm white. White people can't dance. We can only make fools of ourselves while holding our drink and thinking sipping it is hiding the missing rhythm.

"Bartender, can I get six more shots please?!"

Introductions and embrace-filled handshakes all around. Her soft touch moved my eyes from our hands to her gentle smile. Southern beauty. A smile turned shiver as my mind silenced to a mumbling "hello." Frozen in the moment, saved by the whiskey. The mood eased. We drank, we laughed, we talked, we got drunk, and we danced…glass in hand. On the brightest note, for once my bowels didn't ruin the moment. On the saddest note, alcohol did. "Hope to spee you again," I slurred. Much to my delight, she agreed as her eyelids fell, head dropped, and she crashed to the floor.

"Check please," exclaimed my roommate.

Leaving with empty wallets and a tilted sway, our obnoxious excitement met breakfast cravings for the Wiffle Mouse. Waddle Health. Wiffle Blouse. Pitchers, shots, and well whiskey are a gut-eating hell of a punch. "Yes, can I have the cheese 'n' eggs with bacon and hash browns smothered, covered, peppered, and chunked? And a large orange juice? Shank you. Thank mew. Ah…" The best orders are ingrained in the unconscious mind.

What do you mean I am going to now drunkenly eat and get increasingly annoyed with every easily misunderstood statement? Slurred speech turned to tension and inarticulate arguments. My thoughts and confusion about my sickness often came out in the release of intoxication, followed by the walk home's somber honesty. "Nobody understands the pain I'm living with, man. All I hear is how sensitive and annoying I am. I'm in pain and nobody gets that."

Except my bed and the sheets that tuck us away. To that bed I collapsed. Product returned. Same as before. Just another day.

Walk through the routines of that day. We all live in some form of the day's truth. The food, the irresponsibility, hiding from failure, masking to just get by, or altering our state to temporarily forget about the pain. All of that finds us at one time or another. The circumstances may be different, but the habits remain and adjust to the same. I stumbled through that sad reality for over a decade, ignoring and running from its truths. "You only live once" was my repeated phrase of justification. The positives were present and healing was always there. Unfortunately, the laughingly accepted lifestyle blinded any chance for positive change.

During this time in college, another conversation included the recommendation of drinking milk to alleviate the growing severity of a painful abdominal cramping episode. I drank the milk without doing due diligence first. By nighttime, I was sweating profusely, having squeezing diarrhea, and curled in bed from the stabbing pain. Luckily, someone who cared, the dancer-turned-girlfriend, was by my side to persuade the reluctance of going to the emergency room. Diagnosis: severe dehydration. A few weeks later there was another episode and a dart-at-the-wall solution of two weeks of Cipro.

That was it. No other suggestion of underlying cause. No connections or concerns. Not the fact that my diet was…well, you can piece that together. Not the fact that I was losing most of everything I put in and was depleting my body to the point of dehydration. Nor the back pain that, at this time, radiated with each episode's draining. Nor even looking into the repeated patterns of my mental wellbeing. That ambulance ride wasn't from asthma or a bleeding rectum. It was from a defeated and broken mind that hadn't been fed correctly for almost two decades.

Again, an ailment was masked with a treatment while the root cause carried on running its operation. Like arresting the drug dealers while never looking for the supplier. The yellow muck in my stool was acidic bile being flushed from my stomach because the agitation throughout the digestive tract triggered a stoppage of work and the irritants opened the valve until every last drop was gone. I was losing all fluids before they could properly be used to run the body efficiently, which led to dehydration and was irritated further by an overdose of dairy. Not an insufficient consumption of water.

How about the answer for the dull-turned-sharp throbbing that had now moved from the abdomen to the very ends of my digestive tract? A family doctor had the diagnosis: prostatitis.

Prostatitis. The newest dart in this game of blind bullseye. "Can you just take the pain away, Doc?" Request received. Diagnosis fulfilled. Antibiotics prescribed. Plan continued. Again.

This draining only grew more confusion, sadness, depression, and deprivation in the already deprived. Time passed and I went to doctors and therapists. They explained my symptoms and helped figure out...well, nothing. I was extensively tested and treated for each ailment. Overall, I wasn't getting any better. I was coping. The ability to link each illness and symptom had yet to develop. The extent of the attack on my body couldn't be understood. The internet was a scary place with perplexing, generalized answers that led to more fear than resolve. Leading to overusing and easily trusting.

Another issue, similar to the blind prescribing of that day's events, was Adderall. Every era has a substance that spreads like a virus. Some substances are shamefully renamed and reintroduced, like amphetamines. We can test for nutrient deficiencies, broken bones, or cancer, but the diagnosis of this particular "disease," ADD, is solely up to the discretion of a health care professional, who has been shaped and guided by who knows what influences or motives or education. Which increases the need to self-advocate and make decisions after having explored the entire spectrum of knowledge.

Although I was never diagnosed as ADD or ADHD, I was often told I was because of my nonstop talking and outbursts of "unusual" energy. I mean, everyone at that time was in one way or another an ADD candidate. Having seen the epidemic and controlling nature of the drug, that was one I was happy to have missed out on. I used it on occasion, but the fact I was not prescribed it avoided pulling me into the dangers of its "been up six days straight" addiction.

With Adderall surprisingly missing from my drug cocktail, I lovingly accepted Xanax, Tylenol, oxycodone, Xanax, inhalers, Mucinex, Prednisone, Pepto, Benadryl, antibiotics, whiskey, and on and on, all part of surviving my day by constantly putting out fires that were wearing me and my relationships thin. Growing up, I could manage some sort of balance because I was active and young. But by now, it was withering. Everything I was losing and masking by recklessly ignoring was taking over, and my only sanctuaries were comedy, alcohol, drugs, and isolation. Misunderstood's confusing hideout and depression's weight room. My loneliness lived with the fluctuations and persistent diagnoses of ailments and disease. Until Memorial Day weekend of my last summer in college, when the pain reached new heights and the disease finally grew a name.

CHAPTER 6: Diagnosis

Life is so unpredictably predictable. A girlfriend's father once told me, "You can't live and hide through your bad habits forever. Life always catches up with you." He was referring to himself and his lifetime of poor health and choices, I think. Regardless, he was right. You can only outrun and mask your health and bad habits for so long before they catch up and reveal the damage. At that point, your only hope is that it's something you can recover from. Living through the game of knowing it's coming and ignoring the extent of what it'll be is like playing Russian roulette. Except the gun is fully loaded and your survival lies in the severity of the bullet.

According to a study conducted by the National Center for Health Statistics at the Centers for Disease Control and Prevention, "the average body weight of both sexes rose 25 pounds between the years of 1960 and 2002." Twenty-five pounds to our added reality. The mind immediately leaps to the answer: our food. Our food is a major contributor, a culprit, in our reckless lifestyles. Nevertheless, it's not the complete answer. The world has sped up remarkably since 2002, exponentially since 1960, and only faster as we move forward, constantly evolving to improve efficiency for the easiest life possible. That's the goal. Enjoy the furthest reaches of existence in the most comfort for the short time you are blessed with it. Which is why our diseases are not just one thing, they're everything put in our way for us to happily consume in the belief that it isn't affecting us. Our habits, toxic loads, food quality, and lifestyles drag us along while adding those pounds and keeping us from fulfilling a healthy promise to ourselves. Maybe it is set up for our failure. Maybe it's not. How you view it through the madness is the difference. That's the simple change.

On Christmas Eve in 1992, just before dusk, I remember my mom frantically rushing around our house barking orders as we ignored her, and Dad waited outside our thawing-out suburban, smoking a cigarette. Every family has, or should have, a tradition. At that time in our lives, it was Christmas Eve at Grandpa and Grandma Selge's. We were our standard thirty minutes late. It was Mom's fault, always. It's not like she wasn't cooking all day, wrapping presents, ironing, and making sure her youngest didn't burn the house down, all while getting ready with curlers in her hair and yelling at four boys to get dressed. (That still includes one grown man.) There are no days off for a mom. Especially not around the holidays.

When we finally arrived at their front door, my brother grabbed the knob. It was locked. My dad didn't believe him or find the joke funny. It was cold. "Open the door." He then reached out for himself, and said, "Marv's door is never locked. Ring the bell." We shivered while waiting patiently for someone to come, when all of a sudden, "Pop, pop, pop, pop!" Instant terror. A pack of firecrackers landed beside Mom. After pulling our hearts from the frozen asphalt we all looked up to see Grandpa leaning out of his kitchen window, holding his pipe and letting out a hollering laugh that only a lifelong smoker can capture. "Don't drop the baked beans, sweetie!"

The baked beans are a prized family recipe that fell to my mother's responsibility, and she never let expectations down even when also preparing pistachio pudding, a cheese ball, and kieflies cookies. My aunts divided the deviled eggs, three bean salad, jello mold, and cheesy potatoes. Grandma prepared the ham and turkey, mashed potatoes, stuffing, and pumpkin pie. Traditional dishes, detrimental combinations, overloaded amounts. Toxins, dairy, allergies, wrong fats, processed this, sugar rush that, and so on and simple changes detailed later. All washed down with Grandpa's iconic punch—that I ate the fruit of out for years without knowing the toxicity for me of each melon ball. His special punch loosened the mood for a night of embrace and appreciation, letting go of all else the year holds.

The cuckoo clock popped its head, sounding the top of the hour with an annoying chirp, and Grandma finished the buffet with sliced honey ham. My mom yelled from the top of the steps for my brothers. "Boys! Dinner's ready!" The family lined the table in their usual positions, in order of age, descending down to the kids' side fold-out table where I happily ate dinner with my younger cousins well into my teens. Grandpa usually passed the wine with an adult joke that brought out a laugh for himself and mixed reactions from the ones who understood.

This year, I remember standing next to him to ask a question, and the movement of that frame stopping to the watching faces of everyone down the table. Of the thirteen adults looking back, nine eventually suffered from either cancer, chronic pain, or debilitating illness. The oldest, Mee-Maw, was the healthiest. She lived to be ninety-six, and her dad nearly the same. Knowingly damaging their body or not, their frames withstood life's overcrowded expedition for a reason. Happy people, in a happy time. To that, Grandpa blessed the table with a raise of his wine and his appropriate toast. "Over the lips, through the tongue, look out stomach, here I come!"

After dinner, our rotating Santa would unload the presents from under the tree. The toys played, the adults laughed, and the punch drained. As a kid, the concept of time and structure of life has yet to develop.

Time shrinks with age, a perception that is only understood by living more of it. There's no other period in life that has more meaning than the fractions you get to spend with your family, or the ones who feel like family. Better health, more days.

That pipe my Grandpa Selge was holding while hanging out of that window in 1992 was his end in 1996. Mouth cancer that spread to no recovery. That Christmas Eve was the last healthy memory of our tradition. He missed all my sports, our milestones, vacations, births, and weddings. He missed my brother's wedding in 2007, when I spent one of the days hungover, watching a movie with my niece before another night of tending bar. We shared a bag of raw broccoli and ranch. A deadly good combination.

"Uncle Brandon, what's in ranch?" her eight-year-old innocence asked.

"Something we probably shouldn't be eating," while dipping and consuming another round.

"Isn't broccoli good for us though?" They absorb everything, good and bad.

"Yes, and that's why we should eat the whole bag!" Empty bag, empty bottle, bad habits passed on.

That night, while I was tending the bar, perfecting margaritas, I started feeling the usual bloating cramp in my abdomen. I worked through it, thinking the routine was in motion and the gas would pass. As the pain worsened, my mom lovingly dropped off the Pepto-Bismol. I was able to fight it off for a couple more hours, until the point I could barely stand. This had developed into the worst pain I had ever felt. Worse

61

than any other cramping, broken bones, flus, or wounds. This was something different. I left work mid-rush and drove to the ER, having to pull over twice from this "new evolution's" near blackout.

At first, the doctors believed my appendix had burst. They were not entirely certain what was happening, therefore they could not administer any sort of pain medication. The pain was coming and going, each tightening heightening the intensity. It took a little under an hour before the doctor gave the order to administer pain medication. An hour that slowed to the pace of eternity.

I was back. Hotel de Hospital. Finally being forced to figure out what had been plaguing me for so long. After the appendix issue had been ruled out and tests had been run, the doctors were still unable to make a final diagnosis. They sent me home after a couple of days, and after a few weeks of prescribed antibiotics, steroids, and procedures, I remember my new gastroenterologist coming into the examination room with confused determination and saying, "Well, I finally know your diagnosis. Crohn's disease. An intestinal issue where ulcers form in a certain part of your colon and disrupt the digestive tract."

Well, there we go. After all this time. What I now know as a "flare-up" is common for Crohn's disease. This also taught me my first food lesson with my now-named condition. Raw food like broccoli agitates Crohn's disease and triggers intestinal flare-ups. The mystery ingredients in a bottle of ranch dressing didn't help.

The doctor then went on to say, "I don't know a lot about it, but we're going to learn about this thing together." Yeah, no thanks. The next day we scheduled an appointment at the University of Chicago

Medical Center, with one of the best-known specialists in the country. "The guy" for Crohn's disease. As nice as that first doctor was—and I'm all for learning curves—I was not about to "learn about this thing together." When it comes to our personal survival you reach as far as you can, never settling for anything less. That's another responsibility we owe ourselves. Quick side note: How many prescriptions for antibiotics and steroids do you think I'd been given up to this point? Somewhere in the thirties, probably.

There I was. Newly diagnosed with Crohn's disease. That explains everything. Wait, what *is* Crohn's disease? Does it go away? Is there a cure? Will I die? I'm twenty-two years old and want to live the same life a normal twenty-two-year-old should live. The only answers we had at that point were a trifold pamphlet from Doctor Learn-about-This-Thing-Together, an appointment, and the scariest of suggestions from the internet. Like having my intestine cut out or colon cancer or lymphoma. Life-ending possibilities. I was relieved that maybe we were finally on to something, and terrified because of not knowing what that something entailed.

After having gone down the rabbit hole of my health for a little over two decades, pulling up to the Chicago Medical Center reassured us all that I was going to finally get some relief. Checking-in's patience with never-ending forms led us to vitals and then to the examining room for our saving grace's arrival. He introduced himself, went over my records, and talked at great length, explaining everything to expect and understand about where we were and what was ahead.

"This is a genetics-based disease. Unfortunately, there is no cure. It's tough to manage, and even harder to put into remission."

We were confident the plan he laid out would be a route to remission and all that was needed was watching the progress. From there, I was put on my first medicine for the disease: Pentasa. Along with a few other usual suspects like a steroid, nausea meds, another antibiotic, and an anti-inflammatory pill. A colonoscopy was ordered, and I was to come back and see him the week after. While leaving, the doctor looked at my dad, shook his hand, and assured him he was "our doctor for life."

That was the last day I saw Doctor For-Life. At twenty-two, I was no longer eligible for my parents' insurance. Still having one more semester of college and now a "pre-existing condition," I was denied insurance. Because of being uninsured and paying cash, I never saw anyone more than his assistant again. I don't blame him. It's the way the system goes. This was on me, the one who should've taken it into his own hands and explored other options to figure out solutions. But that kind of understanding takes years. You can build the shiniest medical tower with gold toilets and diamond elevators, but it's all a piece in the game that is our second decade of the twenty-first-century mismanaged health care system. You walk through those doors. They don't walk through you.

The insurance issue and extreme prices brought doctor-approved bulk-ordered medicine from Canada. Seven times cheaper and a wholesale of thousands. Mixed with the rest of the crew, I was taking numerous pills a day and back to living. Except, from now on, living with a diagnosis. Crohn's disease.

When you're convinced medicine is the sole solution for this "genetic-based" autoimmune condition, there isn't much need to face habits and addictions. The solution was so easy. Too good to be true. This was all I had to do all along? These pills?

Let this be the lesson: Limited opinions breathe a tunneled vision, and tunnel vision directs naïve choices. Nevertheless, I had an answer, and I started living and breathing it.

CHAPTER 7: Life's Change

There are periods of life, short or long, near or far, that seem like lifetimes ago. There are people who come, people who go, and people left in the mind of a time. College and she are my mind's time, lifetimes ago. She and I experienced the first freedom of life, together. In love. Hundreds of versions of myself have been shed since those years. The good and bad thing about first love is the understanding you gain for the next time it comes. Unfortunately, that doesn't secure its forever promise. Love comes to the available and stays with the ready. Then, and only then, it grows with you. Habits and health do the same. Regrettably, until we're ready for anything, we're going to lose along the way. It's inevitable. Family, friends, disease, control, jobs, auditions, endless loss through the growing of time and the growing of existence. The only thing that cannot be lost twice is our life, and until we are surrounded by the healthiest version of ourselves, she will let go. Unfulfilled and into the land of what if and forever left lifetimes ago.

I graduated college. A complete shock to everyone. I wasn't ever on the dean's list and barely ever in "good standing." Regardless, as a reward for the accomplishment, I took the winter off to figure out my next steps. A newly graduated bachelor with a degree in Logistics. Cincinnati, Atlanta, trucking, shipping? Questions. Important life decisions. I have a great degree in something I love, now let's build with it. The problem with that was, it wasn't honest. I had never found any appeal in the idea of working for a company, for a lifetime, doing repetitive tasks and riding off into the retirement sunset. I've always known there was a unique meaning for my path. Maybe yours is the aforementioned because it provides your life with something else. "Do

I like doing concrete work? No, it's hard. But it provides everything I want for the rest of my life and my family. That's more important to me," my dad told me once. Mine rotates in another fashion. Same satisfaction, different vision.

The problem at that time was, what was next? Even many years later, today as I'm writing, I'm still stressing that very question. Dad, again, has also repeatedly reassured me over the years: "I'm this age and I still don't know what I want to do. Stop worrying about it. Just do." Coming from a man who has worked hard to successfully own and operate several businesses over his lifetime, all while skillfully playing his harmonica and being good at darts and pool. Our stubbornly matched egos aside, he is right. Step into the changes you've always wanted to make, and be comfortable with them while becoming a new version of yourself.

During the winter of 2007, I chose to go home. My parents' new home. On the shores of Lake Michigan, just over the state line from Indiana, lies an amiable beach town that swells three times in size during the summer months and deserts into bundled solitude with the howls of Lake Michigan's winter freeze, when throwing hot water on your car windshield replaces the chilly strain of repeatedly scraping and chipping away a layer of ice. Summer's beach vibes huddle around a cozy fire, heater, or the expedient atmosphere of a locally enriched coffee shop. Childhood chocolate milk and donuts replaced by adult bagels, muffins, and freshly brewed coffee. Too often, we don't realize the wealth that periods of our lives give us until the seizing of it has long gone. I gained the appreciation of the in-between times, from this time.

By mid-April, it was clear. My childhood friend and I had decided. We were going to pursue our sixth-grade dream and take our college degrees across the country. We were moving to Los Angeles. No fear. Just optimism at the thought of infinite opportunity. Neither of us had ever been there before. Nonetheless, in mid-September we would go, or "just do." From that decision, my perfect margaritas and fajitas of the previous summer shifted to martinis and upscale Italian. I worked hard, partied harder (because that's the cliché healthy phrase, right?), stuck with my unconscious habits, consumed healthy amounts of Pentasa, compiled sock drawer dollars, and as the summer turned to September, departed. Looking back, the decision was immensely bold and a now-proud retrospect of my life. No stopping, no second guessing, just doing.

One failure, that I will humbly admit as a failure, was failure to take my health into consideration. It was an afterthought and rightfully so, since that's the space of mind it had always occupied. At that point I was committed to the Pentasa plan for the Crohn's and was just starting to understand things like gluten and raw broccoli being triggers for a flare-up, a flare-up that the plan was supposed to calm, and so I justified my way to happily suffering through drinking beer and overindulging in pizza. Even though I knew better.

With health assuming the back-seat position, realization of a period's end struck.

"This isn't bye, it's see you soon," I said to my mother.

"We're always here," she squeezed back.

"You be good," said my dad with rare emotion. A phrase I had heard his father tell him during my youth and he now chokingly passed on to me.

Bittersweet at its sweetest bitterness. Never thinking that home would ever change, we left on our cross-country excursion, traveling to friends in Lincoln, Nebraska and camping in the Rocky Mountains. From bars in Fort Collins to a lady in New Mexico. Hiking Sedona, stumbling through Vegas, and welcomed by the every-hour traffic of the 101 freeway. Pentasa popped, whiskey flowed, and fast food filled our stomachs. After seventeen days of the greatest trip a new adult could take, we were home. In the city of angels. Los Angeles, California.

First moments found a corner booth at Denny's on Sunset Boulevard, enjoying chicken strips and cheese fries. We ate to the accomplishment of our trip and ended our lunch to the reality of not having prepared anything beyond this point.

"Ok, now what?"

We didn't have any friends, housing, jobs, or idea of where to start.

"How about the Chinese Theater?"

We were determined to get here, and we did.

"Let's do Venice Beach!"

The rest was lost in the excitement of having the balls to actually take the leap.

"The Hollywood sign?"

But, like everything else in life, "just do," and let the rest present itself.

"Beverly Hills and Rodeo Drive it is!"

Stepping outside the box is a scary place and often gets disregarded by the fearful justification of not knowing what's next. Contained life never seeks the growth in healthier opportunity.

Four days later, our lack of credit, jobs, and anything suitable to allow normal tenancy found a small basement apartment just over the hill from Hollywood in Studio City, or "the valley," where the stereotypical landlord grumpily monitored our moves and a picture window overlooked a beautifully built concrete wall. The kind only a concrete man like my dad would appreciate. Everyone else, not so much. Sunlight? Not so bright. Regardless, we made it a home. Rent that would normally provide months of luxury anywhere else found us a floor underground decorated with furniture plucked from the sidewalks or hauled through the thrift store. It didn't matter. We were here, and our place slowly filled while we adjusted to our new life. I slept on a double thick queen air mattress and feasted on boxed mac 'n' cheese, cheap spaghetti, and the liquor store special of the week.

Eventually we found jobs, and for the next several months settled in. Except the jobs proved to be unsettling. Remember that job in college with great people, exciting work, and perks? Those days were long gone. Enter everyday stress that compiled and offered limited opportunity for advancement. Extreme anxiety and on-the-edge stress wear down your immune system. Mix that with stalled progress and an appetite for low-quality food, and a "healthy" contribution to disease you will make. At that point, we had to move forward by moving on to something else. Except my friend was moving back. Meaning, it was just me and the few friends I had made in the short time of being there. We lost our apartment. I bounced around, couch surfing, trying to find my place. Searching for another job. I knew I wasn't going back to Michigan. I had made the choice to explore a change and I was determined to give it a legitimate shot. Even though I had little money left and was hiding in the shadows of a disease that was taking me closer to death, I knew there was something there for me to find.

Stress, lifestyle, diet, Pentasa, inhaler, no exercise, and days of nervous anxiety were all covered with comedic hiding that provoked me to finally leap into my childhood dream: acting. I had taken a few classes in college, developed skills as a videographer, and had a passion for editing. That lead to enrolling in a school that taught the methods of Sanford Meisner and a quietly cool back-alley theater for improv classes, completing a balance of freedom in an acting method and the open interpretation of improvisation. This was the plan my friend and I dreamed up in the sixth grade.

I was now living on a twin air mattress in the living room of my first friend in LA and his exuberantly happy, much older roommate's never-cleaned apartment and working as a server while taking classes. Despite the hours of release the acting classes provided, I was still hiding in the darkest spaces life offers at every opportunity. Dwelling in the unresolved.

From there, my drugs added other drugs, routinely, to get away from reality and get relief from the lost appetite and extreme nausea that plagued most of my days. I'd get six or seven tacos and substance abuse my confusion into oblivion on a back street in the heart of "the valley." Then walk through the front door to the dirt-thick, mold-encrusted living room of a substance-abused apartment. The friendly environment that invited the decision to join, had in just months dissipated into the lost of my friend's addiction and his girlfriend's influence. I didn't know they were doing what they were doing. They were my friends and kept it to themselves. That time slowly wore him away into a shell of the person I first met. He hid in the deadly addiction until one evening when a fight broke out in his bedroom with a couple of "visitors." My reaction from the intense stress of that evening was an abdomen that sent crippling pain and a downward spiral that had gone ignored for a lifetime too long.

As that girlfriend's father once said, "Life always catches up to you." Well, it did.

CHAPTER 8: The House Collapses

DATE OF ADMISSION: 05/04/2010

HISTORY OF PRESENT ILLNESS: The patient is a 25-year-old male with a past medical history significant for Crohn's disease. The patient presents to the ER per recommendation of his new IBD specialist. The patient reports that over the past several weeks he has had increased abdominal pain, nausea without vomiting, fever, and diaphoresis. He has also noted increased severity of his diarrhea from a baseline of less than 3 bowel movements a day to 10-20 bowel movements a day which awakens the patient at night due to the urgency. The patient says that there has not been any significant blood noted in the bowel movements, although bloody bowel movements have been a feature of his disease in the past. The patient also notes that he has had a significant amount of bloating in the abdomen. The abdominal pain that he notes is located mostly in the right lower quadrant, is sharp, and has no clear precipitants or alleviating factors. The patient reports that these symptoms started worsening approximately 5 weeks ago. He increased his dose of Pentasa; he normally takes approximately 6 tablets a day and increased this to approximately 12-14 tablets a day. The patient reports that he will often do this when he has a Crohn's flare and this usually resolves his symptoms. However, this time around he did not have resolution of his symptoms. The patient reports that this is a particularly bad flare for him. He has noted a 11-pound weight loss which is something that he has not experienced in the past. The pain and the degree of diarrhea are also more severe than he has had with prior flares. In the ER the patient was given 2 liters of normal saline and 2 mg of Dilaudid.

REVIEW OF SYSTEMS: *Positive for hip and left leg and lower back pain. The patient reports that the pain has been present since his teenage years, and the back pain is something that he does not usually feel when he has the Crohn's flare. He denies any other joint pain, rashes, or visual changes.*

REASON FOR ADMISSION: *Crohn's flare*

Sooner or later we are all forced to take responsibility for our irresponsibility. Sadly, and all too often, we take responsibility when it "catches up" to us. The night of the drug-induced brawl, I packed up and left. My friend and his girlfriend vanished. For years I thought they had died or he had been murdered or was in jail or whatever other thought crosses your mind through losing connection like that. The problem with the incident was, it pushed me over the edge. My health had now gone too far and was too exposed. I went home to get away and be with family, then came back a week later to find a new apartment and new peace.

Unfortunately, not even the royal palace was going to save me this time. The only thing masking my decline was THC and oxycodone, and often. For nausea, for lost appetite, for pain, for depression, and for ignoring already exposed lungs. I was high more often than I wasn't. Weeks grew and pain overcame the situation. When I drove myself to the hospital for the "appendix bursting" incident, I had waited minutes too long and was a danger behind the wheel. That attack was suffered due to several weeks of being too stubborn in the thought of not having insurance or a way to pay for a hospital visit, and grown from decades of…well, yeah. A sad situation to put oneself in.

A flare-up like that, or of any kind, exposes you to the sudden chaos of an immune system that proliferates any existing condition, from ulcers, fistulas, abscesses, and inflammation along the entire digestive tract. The environment is battered, weakened, and unstable. Symptoms vary depending on location, and severity comes with the progression of unmanaged damage. In this case, when the colon is under attack the cells multiply and intense inflammation allows harmful chemicals and bacteria into the intestinal walls, causing the entire colon to flush—diarrhea—accompanied by bloating, nausea, fatigue, poor appetite, mucus/bile loss, ulcers, fevers, and depression. All the major effects of an immune system attacking itself while inflammation, yeast overgrowth, bad bacteria, parasites, and infection obstruct and happily expand. Remember, 80 percent of the immune system resides in the gut, and these symptoms are general for many conditions. Given the pain patterns and location, mixed with the combination of increasingly worsening debilitating symptoms, I was having an intestinal flare-up.

Twenty bowel movements a day. Tiny burning squeezing throughout the digestive tract emptying to the last drop, clammy sweats, and aching lack of energy are a few effects of compromised immunity and fractured intestinal lining. Resulting in eleven pounds lost in a month, crippling pain, and limited options while remaining blindly naïve and carelessly ignoring all possibilities that could cause such pain. Twenty-five years with a diseased body creates a comfort in the irresponsibility of taking fourteen pills a day as a lame attempt at maintaining optimal health and ignoring the voice in the back of the mind that is screaming that the problem is growing out of control. Falsely convincing myself that the "remission plan," or maintenance plan, was the solution. Immediate relief becomes the necessity, and I'm left in an urgent situation of driving to the ER for the first major flare-up since diagnosis. Bring out the blue slippers and buttocks-revealing gown, I'm back.

HOSPITAL COURSE:

The patient was admitted in stable condition to the Medicine Teaching Service. The patient had been evaluated by the IBD team while in the emergency room and was initiated on IV Solu-Medrol at 20 mg every 8 hours. The patient was also continued on his Pentasa orally. The patient's pain was controlled with Vicodin as needed, and he was given IV fluids for hydration as he had some mild evidence of acute kidney injury likely due to dehydration.

The patient had significant improvement in his abdominal pain on the day of discharge. He also did not have any loose bowel movements during his admission. Upon further evaluation by the IBD team, the patient was found to be stable for discharge and is to follow-up as an outpatient with the IBD Service Clinic.

FINDINGS:

KUB showing no obstruction or perforation/free air.

(*NOTABLE BLOOD WORK RESULT)

Component:

C-Reactive Protein

Value:

17.5

Reference Range:

<0.80 MG/DL

Flag:

H

CONDITION ON DISCHARGE: Stable

DATE OF DISCHARGE: 05/05/2010

This was diagnosed as a "routine" flare-up and with routine comes routine treatment. Treatment for dehydration and pain resulted in a one-night stay at the five-star hospital of Creme de la Creme. That was all that was needed to bring the patient back to a stable condition and be on his way. My way. The instant solution's comfort had calmed the fire. Immediate relief medicine, a new GI doctor, new living conditions, and revived energy were the courses of action to remission. Unfortunately, the pilot to the already existing monster was still well lit. When it becomes a part of your life to go, get the relief, and go on, you become blind to anything outside of the standard box. A method that allows falling back into comfortable routines led to this moment and will continue to progress once the lethal antibiotic hoses stop spraying.

In all honesty, I knew I wasn't better. I felt it. Something was still wrong. The silver lining was, I established a connection with a new GI doctor who was good and whose educated demeanor brought a trust and respect you want with your doctor. Any doctor. Unsettled were my thoughts of how am I going to pay for the visit, stay, release, and everything between? Through the guidance of the hospital I collected numerous personal documents, filled out forms, and applied for every available charity and program. Decisions were pending.

From the combination of medicines, I was stable. Not healing. Stable and working a new solution while keeping the same course. The steroids had me angry, mentally withdrawn, tired, depressed, and removed from the outside world. Because there was still something churning. Thoughtlessly, I went back to masking, comedy, class, socializing, boxed mac 'n' cheese, and all the usual suspects that so happily filled my tormented reality. I would still wake up to a bowl of marshmallow-anything cereal and end the day the same. Grabbing beers after class with classmates. Stoned fast food. Pizza Fridays. Stress eating. Celebration toasting. You only live once justifications. A monster to the body and fun party to the world. Living on for a month. Growing away from "stable."

DATE OF ADMISSION: 06/02/2010

Patient began experiencing some discomfort in his abdomen yesterday by 9 p.m. and he began having diarrhea with fever. He describes several episodes of dark bloody stools associated with diarrhea. He drank coffee and went to bed in the middle of the night and woke up with chills. This morning, he had an additional 6 episodes of diarrhea. In fact, he felt so unwell that upon going to the bathroom, he had a syncopal episode. He has no (current) vomiting but he feels nauseated. He complains of diffuse abdominal discomfort.

The patient also complains of right shoulder pain. He has been experiencing this pain since Saturday. The pain does not vary with movement. He denies any fall or trauma or strenuous activity. He has no cough. He does advocate worse with deep breathing.

CURRENT MEDICATIONS: 1. Zosyn. 2. Prednisone 50 mg daily. 3. Pentasa

ADMITTING DIAGNOSIS: Crohn's flare versus infectious diarrhea

"I just want to sleep a little more and I'll feel better," I told my mom. "Brandon. Go to the ER," she replied. Lost in a mind captured by disease: "No! I don't have insurance and this is my own fault anyways." Her motherly tone shifted from pleading to strong: "I'm calling an ambulance." Elevating louder and stubborn in the thoughts that mean nothing to living and being healthy, "NO! I won't be able to pay for it!" Not taking no for an answer: "I'll call Tre then. Give me his number."

The night before, while playing in the now-old-man's softball league, I grabbed a routine grounder in the outfield and went to throw it to second base. Upon release, my entire body went numb. Tingling from fingers to chest. The ball landed halfway and I went lifeless on the dark grass. My world went to the brink of black and was brought back by the calls of teammates around the field. Through the distorted blur: "Brandon, are you ok?" I lifted to grasp the significance of what just happened, and a throbbing in my back-right shoulder radiated with every breath and was accompanied by a stabbing pain inside the right-side torso. "I'm good. Just some shoulder pain." Life's hardening of past illnesses and years of outsiders' doubtful comments taken to heart develops mulishness about taking the logical course of action. We feel we need to be strong versus the reality of what we feel within.

I don't remember drinking coffee. But in a delusional state like that, I don't doubt something justified it. What I do remember was the vomiting was far worse than a one-episode affair. I had been taken lightly on my first ER visit, and as hours passed, thoughts of just working through this severe flare-up and attempting to calm with water and sleep slowly shifted through the night to losing hope. *This was my fault in the first place. It's how it ends. It's what I deserve.*

Struggling to peel off the bed for something as simple as a sip of water brought agonizing pain and sharp bathroom rushes. From bed to toilet was only a few steps, but blurred vision from the loss of fluids grew the distance as my sweaty stagger faded in and out of consciousness. The toilet painted red from my body's leaking of blood. Crawling back brought on extreme nausea and the water from minutes prior found the overflowing bucket by the bed. With every trip, my clothes slowly colored red and soaked in sweat. Throughout the night my thoughts and body weakened. The pain worsened. The symptoms became more debilitating. I accepted the end. Justified by my own failures. I was ok with dying there, because it was better than suffering another day.

"Tre, Brandon is in bad shape. He won't let us call 911. He's locked in his room. Can you check on him?" Without hesitation, my new classmate dropped what he was doing and ran three miles from house to apartment where he and my roommate picked their way into the bedroom and to their shock found my rail-thin body unresponsive on the bed. The severity of the situation took hold and they lifted me, placed me in my car, and Tre drove like a crazy taxi over the hill into Beverly Hills to my new GI's office. "You ok, man?" No response. "Brandon?" He pulled to the building's curb and sprinted inside for help. My next moments of presence came with the collective effort of my doctor, his assistant, and Tre laying me on an office table. The doctor checked my vitals and I answered his questions with mumbles. Moving his examination over my abdomen, he listened and pressed different locations. Eventually striking the spot and wakening a moment of presence with a piercing scream. Fearful about my condition, the doctor ordered, "Get him to the ER! I'll let them know you're coming."

After Tre Andretti frantically wheeled me to the ER, an hour passed before I was admitted and placed on a gurney in the emergency room's hallway. An hour of severe contraction-like convulsions heightened the agonizing depths of radiating shoulder pain. Tre nervously waited in a chair at the end of my bed. Another hour passed. Nobody came. Another hour. Nothing. He stopped a nurse. "Excuse me, is anyone going to help my friend? He's in bad shape!" She looked back at him as if we were nothing. No insurance and "mild attack" assumptions led to this. Treatment limited because of the lack of something I could never gain in the first place from a "pre-existing condition." Admitted because of my current condition, not treated because of the system and postulation of it being, as one nurse put it, "just another flare-up."

That's when a doctor passed. Through my disillusioned weakness, I grabbed his jacket as he went by. He stopped. I pleaded. "Please help me. Don't let me go. Something's wrong." He compassionately grabbed my hand and while checking me over, said, "You don't look well. I promise I won't until I figure out what's wrong." That doctor's understanding and willingness to help saved my life.

At his orders, the same nurse administered a shot of morphine directly into my arm a few minutes later. The warm tingle from the injection travelled down my spine and provided the most relieving delight that would make any opioid addict smile. Four hours in, and four hours later, I woke up on that same bed in the same hallway. I had yet to be moved into a room or taken for any scans. Lack of insurance was still finding a solution. I glanced to the end of the bed and in a hospital chair, there was napping Tre. Another four hours passed until they finally moved me into a curtain-divided space. "Tre, please go, man. You've done more than I could ever ask for." At that point, he had stayed a total of twelve hours. He missed work, class, and his life to be there. For a friend. No matter how bad we feel in this world, good shows up when all else fails. Everyone says they'll be there but, in the end, few do and I'm grateful he did. That's the real in life. Money is made up, insurance is made up, but friends like him are the substance.

During the time from my mom's plea and finally being admitted into a room, my dad again dropped everything and drove the two hours to Chicago, found a flight, and arrived in LA by nightfall. He and I were in the hospital room the next day when a man came in and introduced himself as the lead doctor of what would eventually be a team of doctors for my case. He said he saw my case on the board, read up on the situation and how I didn't have insurance, and because of his own life's current misfortunes he felt compelled to take it on. His wife had been battling breast cancer and something told him he needed to help here. Regardless of your level of spirituality, this doctor, Dr. Maldonado, was an angel sent to my life when I was on my way out. We talked strategy, life, and solutions. He brought smiles and jokes into the conversation. Nobody knew exactly what was happening to my body. The only thing that was assured was that this was well beyond a routine flare-up. He lined up doctors and tests and guaranteed us that we would find solutions together.

After several days of scans, procedures, tests, dyes, drugs, liquids, and confusion, the doctor came into the room with an answer. He sat in a chair and calmly said, "Well, from the scans, we finally know what

84

it is." His tone turned melancholy. "The problem is, we don't know if we're going to be able to get to it." At that moment my heart sank into the reality and a thousand memories of clouded remorse passed through my mind. Twenty-five years of irresponsible acts developed into that one sentence. I looked at my dad and he had turned solid white. It finally had caught up to me.

INPATIENT RADIOLOGY REPORT

TECHNIQUE: Following the administration of intravenous contrast, spiral CT was performed from the lung bases up through the chest to the level of the apices with timing to optimize maximized opacification of the pulmonary arterial system. Follow this, routine spiral CT was performed from the lung apices down through the chest to the upper abdomen. 2D MIP and 3D angiographic post processing was performed on an independent workstation.

IMAGING STUDIES REPORT

FINDINGS: CT abdomen shows large hepatic abscess in the dome of the liver, approximately 5.1 x 4.1 cm; there is also a potential fistulous tract and several skip lesions noted.

There it is. An abscess on top of the liver. The years of wearing down had forced my immune system into "autoimmunity," and as my army depleted, fighting itself and struggling to keep the enemy from overthrowing my society, the environment grew larger infections, yeast overgrowths, and multiplied the bad bacteria. All while thriving to the beat of the party that was my habitual lifestyle. Eventually the city started to crumble, and as the bacteria ate through my intestinal wall, they widened the gaps for the rest to run rampant into uncharted freedom. There, they latched on to the closest vein and rode the expressway of opportunity to claim a new throne on top of my liver. They invited their family, extended family, neighbors, and that one friend you don't really like but invite anyways because your friend brought him. As the residents arrived, the bubble (abscess) grew and grew and grew. The war may have still been in my gut, but the new colony was on top of my liver. As the population expanded into overpopulation, the abscess began to collapse my lung, causing the shoulder pain.

As the room remained still, I remember thinking, this isn't the end. Not now. I still have so much left to do. I broke the silence by asking the doctor, "How do we solve this?" My dad chimed in. "Is it fatal?" The doctor replied, "We have two options. We can try and find a way to drain the abscess, then heal the exposed parts of your intestines with strong antibiotics, or if we don't feel comfortable with this very risky procedure, we can hope the antibiotics and other medicines close the intestinal exposure and cut off the supply to the abscess. Removal of the infected intestine is a strong possibility, but not an option without healing the abscess first."

At that point it was difficult to even sit up. I had lost so much weight, become so weak, and the pain was so severe that simple movements resulted in a stabbing shock throughout my abdomen, chest, and shoulder. Thankfully, I was heavily medicated. So, what to do? Take the risk, then attack with antibiotics? Or don't take the risk and attack with the same medicines, hoping it'll heal on its own? The doctor spoke up. "I must say, the specialist that would be doing this procedure I know very well, and he's not a gunslinger. If he can get to it, he will. If he has any doubt about it, he won't. But I'll let you guys have some time to talk it out."

The abscess was shielded by my vital organs. Every doctor on my team had a different opinion of how to go about healing it successfully. The problem was, I was at the very edge and one mishap could spiral to the end. At that point in my life, I had had hundreds of doctors for procedures, broken bones, surgeries, ailments, and treatments. None of them projected the confidence I felt from this doctor. My dad agreed. I had left myself with limited options because of being so oblivious to the obvious for so long. What my subconscious had been saying with every bite and sip and stress and neglect had been true.

The doctor came back into the room. We all agreed attempting to drain the abscess was the only option. This was Friday. The procedure was scheduled for Monday night. My mom was home for my cousin's wedding, and my dad and I spent that weekend in my room anxiously passing time. Making the best of the worst. I never doubted this being the end, but I was uneasy of what was about to come. I could see (and smell) the strain in my father by his hiding in his own habits of food and cigars. I wasn't the only one going through this. Irresponsibility brings down our closest as well.

Monday's exiting sun came with the entering of my nurses. "Ready for your procedure?" Did I have a choice? "Of course. Let's get this over with!" We made our way into the room where the procedure would take place. Dim lights lined the edges while one brightly lit light highlighted the obvious. Nurses prepared in the shadows. Dr. Not-Gunslinger came in and introduced himself. "Hi, Brandon. We're going to have a look, and if I see a way, we will drain that abscess. If I don't, we won't. The only thing is, I need you to be fully aware to breathe for me. Meaning, we are going to have to do this without pain medication." Through negotiating, because of the already unbearable pain I was in and the fear I held within, he agreed to give me a small dose of Dilaudid. The only relief it provided was appeasing my overactive mind.

Three nurses lifted me from bed to bed, I held in the tears, we positioned, and he pulled up his chair. The ultrasound machine was hooked up and ready. He applied a cold gel and slowly worked his way around my chest. "We can't go there because of your heart. We can't go there because of the lung. We might be able to go there. We can't do there." He went back over the "we might be able to go there" and decided that is where we could go. "I believe I can successfully reach the abscess by sticking this needle through your liver and inserting a drainage tube attached to this grenade that will slowly suction out the fluids."

The needle was eight inches long.

I nodded and within seconds we proceeded.

06/08/2010:

The patient had CT guided drainage of the liver abscess without complication. The patient experienced some sharp pain after the pigtail catheter was placed, which resolved later that afternoon. A repeat CT abd pelvis (scan) was obtained after the drain was placed, which showed a small collection of blood below the right hemidiaphragm but did not show bleeding at the site of the drain insertion. The drain remained in place and initially collected 10 cc of purulent fluid. Within 24 hours the draining fluid was serosanguinous.

I'll never forget that needle going through my liver. Over the years my diseased body has experienced all aspects of pain. That one stays with me. The bright side was, the procedure worked. I now had a tube running to the abscess and attached to a "grenade" that was successfully suctioning out the fluids. It was not appealing. Red, yellow, white mucus-y pus. Regardless, it was draining, and as we left that room, there was my mom. She had arrived mid-procedure. "Hi, sweetie. We love you, Brandon," they both said while holding my hands. We hadn't told her the severity until the night before. We wanted her to enjoy my cousin's wedding. The happiest times of life. Not where I was.

When I was back in my room, Dr. Maldonado came in. "Well, I'm happy to hear everything went well. Now, we are successfully draining the abscess and I am going to continue to keep you on heavy antibiotics and a variety of other medicines to heal the intestine and abscess while it drains. Then, we will reassess if we need to perform bowel resection surgery."

One large obstacle down, one larger one still lurking.

90

06/10/2010:

The patient improved with the drainage procedure and IV antibiotics. He was able to perform ADLs and was eating a regular diet prior to discharge. Pain controlled was obtained with subQ dilaudid which was transitioned to po Dilaudid once the patient was tolerating po medications.

The patient was evaluated by (the) surgeon for colorectal surgery for future possible surgical intervention of Crohn's disease. No surgery was required during this admission.

Social work and disposition: the patient was approved to receive Charity Care though Cedars-Sinai medical center for his chronic disease management. He was discharged home to receive IV antibiotics for 3 additional weeks (until July 2nd 2010) and will follow up as an outpatient for further management of his Crohn's disease and drain.

CONDITION ON DISCHARGE: Stable

DISCHARGE MEDICATIONS:
1. Flagyl 500 mg orally three times a day.
2. Dilaudid tablet 4 mg orally every 4 hours as needed for pain, #12.
3. Pentasa 1000 mg orally three times a day.
4. Prednisone 12.5 mg by mouth for 7 days, then 10 mg by mouth daily.
5. Rocephin 1 gm intravenously every 24 hours.

DIET: Regular diet

DISCHARGE ACTIVITIES: *Activity as tolerated. The patient was instructed to keep the drain site clean and intact and prevent movement of the drain.*

SPECIAL INSTRUCTIONS: *The patient was instructed to return to the emergency department with worsening abdominal pain, recurrent bloody diarrhea, fevers, chills or pain at the site of the abscess drain or if any complications with the drain arise.*

PROBLEM LIST:

1. Liver abscess

2. Crohn's disease with terminal ileum sinus tract

3. Asthma

The payment uncertainty that prolonged the first trip to the ER and left my body dying before the second, came back with good and bad news. The good news was, one of the programs I applied to accepted me. The bad news was, the remaining private doctor bills and anything done outside of the hospital was to be covered by the patient: me. In this situation the good far outweighed the bad, and with my already obsessed curiosity about every aspect of this process, I was ready for the task. I mean, did I have a choice? The bills that were quickly adding up were real. After eleven days in the hospital, I was pushing six figures. Luckily, the charity I was approved for agreed to cover 100 percent of the hospital bills. Thanks to a deal cut between big tobacco and the government, the same tobacco in the pipe that cost my grandfather his life, eventually gave my dad cancer, and kills nearly 500,000 people in the United States a year, saved my life. I'll never understand how we openly allow everyone to willingly or unwillingly consume or be exposed to the bad but are closed to treating us when we get sick, leaving us scrambling to fight through every loophole possible before expiration.

So, I went home. Home, for now, was an extended stay by the Los Angeles International Airport where my parents had taken up residency for the previous couple of weeks and my mom was a regular with the staff and there was free wine during cocktail hour. Justifiably so. The nurse came on day one, showed us how to administer the hanging antibiotic through my newly inserted PICC line, how to clean the grenade, and how to secure both to prevent infection and the risk of one pulling out (which did slightly happen to the PICC line and caused a quick irregular pulse, accompanied by a fainting feeling). We went over the timing of pills, IV antibiotics, pain meds, and cleanings. Then she was on her way and reality was in the hands of my mom and myself. In that hotel room with boxes of medical supplies and a fridge full of medicine.

I was down thirty-seven pounds since the "brawl" and now had two tubes coming out of my bone-thin body. One from the inside of the left bicep (the PICC line) and one from the middle of my right-side torso (the grenade). Each wrapped tightly with a bandage. Bruises lined my arms from the endless IVs, shots, and stress. All covered by cloths and clothes to save the embarrassment. One great thing was, the pain in my back and my abdomen slowly faded as each day passed. For two weeks, my mom and I lived through the routine of administering and waiting for all to heal.

Despite the stress and the circumstance that brought us together, it was a special two weeks that I will always be grateful to have had with her. We went to the beach, explored Los Angeles, talked, laughed, loved, and enjoyed our time the best we could. Because when life takes you to the brink of death, those rawest moments, presence heightens and nothing else matters other than the time you get with the ones you're with. Life blessed me with great parents and the misfortune blessed us with growth.

During one of our sunny California afternoons, and while enjoying a long lunch at a café on Melrose Avenue, I relished a meal of chili and a healthy juice. As the check came so did another "appendix-bursting" rush. That painful shooting cramp was back. Following doctor's orders, we rushed to the ER. Again, we were back. Again, we waited. Again, we checked into the hospital. Even if I had thought the worst was behind me, here it was.

DATE OF ADMISSION: *06/22/2010 2:31 PM*

CHIEF COMPLAINTS: *Severe abdominal pain*

Pt is alert and oriented. States he is having a severe Crohn's "flare-up" with sharp generalized abdominal pain this am. Skin is warm and dry, color is wnl. Pt's pain comes in waves, rates it 10/10 at this time. Has PICC line in upper arm, and a drain in RUQ which drains from a "liver abscess."

HOME MEDICATIONS:
1. *Prednisone 10 mg daily*
2. *Pentasa 1000 mg t.i.d.*
3. *Flagyl 500 mg t.i.d.*
4. *Dilaudid p.o. 4 mg q.4 hours p.r.n.*
5. *Ceftriaxone IV daily*

HOSPITAL COURSE:
On the first day of hospital admission PT had blood cultures drawn and his IV antibiotics were continued and the colorectal surgery continued to follow the patient. The patient on the second day of hospital admission had a fever of 102 which effervesced. He was on antibiotics and only had mild abdominal pain. He was continued on antibiotics and had pain control and we started discussing possible surgery at that moment.

Before, the doctors debated if my case was a possible infection or a routine flare-up. Then it was whether or not to drain the abscess. Now, it was do we operate and cut out the intestine or continue on heavy antibiotics? Meaning, do we take eighteen inches of colon from this twenty-five-year-old male and leave him with a foot and a half less for the rest of his life, in an area of his body that's crucial to absorbing nutrients? Eighteen inches gone and eighteen inches closer to a colostomy bag.

I was in so much pain that I chose whatever provided a "reset button," and that was surgery. My parents and doctors debated.

The surgeon: "I believe surgery is necessary in this case."

My GI doctor: "Even with surgery it will eventually come back."

The infectious disease doctor: "If you have surgery, the odds of having another surgery are within five years."

My team lead: "Given the state of your condition, I believe surgery is the best choice."

The consensus was in, surgery it was. Five years and a colostomy bag found deaf ears to the immediate condition. A sad reality, in retrospect.

The days leading up to surgery were exhausted by more and more and more procedures and tests. At that point, running a CT scan or similar was becoming less of an option because of the radiation I had already been exposed to. Instead, a chest x-ray was performed to assess the abscess, followed by another procedure that required drinking a liquid to illuminate my organs for a clearer picture. And, eventually, another colonoscopy. Each melting me away a little more, not only physically but mentally too.

For one test, I was taken to a room where they administered the contrasts (fluids) before the procedure. The room felt like it was several stories underground. It was cold, lined with hospital beds filled with people drinking their fluids and getting their IVs, and I was, for the first time, frightened. And weak. And exhausted. And traumatized. The nurse gave me three or four drinks to take over periods of time. I drank and tried to relax and drank and tried again and drank until I couldn't drink anymore. The liquids gurgled. The smell and taste of the mixture was putrid. By the time I got to the end of the second one, another sip wasn't possible. When the next round came, I pleaded with the nurse. "I can't drink this." To which she replied, "You have to. There are no other options." A deep breath, a drink, and vomit. All over myself and my bed. The room turned and the tears rolled through my hands-covered face of shame. My gown was now soaked with everything that was once inside, and my spirit was broken. Sadly, there was a colonoscopy to prep for and a surgery to follow.

Just as with every day, the next day came and I was again given fluids, this time fluids that clean out the system in prep for a colonoscopy. Different day, same worn-thin body still nauseated from the countless ill-tasting drinks and medicines, same worn-thin mind from a lifetime of disease. After the first jug, I curled up in a ball in the corner of the room and refused. I couldn't even speak. Just tears. The doctor was furious and ordered the nurse to administer an enema. I understand now where he was coming from. He needed a clear examination for the surgeon. The nurse came, she administered, I held it in as long as I could and…can we just get to surgery already?

97

FINDINGS:

Colon: *The ileocecal valve was somewhat edematous with some redness around it. With some difficulty, the ileum was intubated and was found to be quite edematous, mildly stenotic and ulcerated. There is a nodularity and serpiginous ulceration throughout the visualized portion of the ileum. There was friability with biopsy. Biopsies were taken in the ileum, cecum, ascending colon, transverse colon, descending colon, sigmoid and the rectum.*

A full fever workup was done for the patient and his antibiotic coverage was broadened to vancomycin and Zosyn. The IBD service was consulted and an upper and lower endoscopy was done which showed nodularity and serpiginous ulceration throughout the ileum. Colorectal surgery was consulted and the patient has now been transferred to the surgery service for ileal resection that is planned for this Tuesday.

Decades of denial now down to this. Cutting the body open, cutting out part of the intestine, sewing it back together, and a fresh start. I was moved to a pre-op suite. Couches, a view of the Hollywood hills and all the necessities for post-surgery. The night before, I lay in that dark room, only illuminated by a red exit sign, with my headphones on, iPod activated (the relic that used to hold our computer-generated song lists on a small digital screen), and my favorite playlist cued. Mixing between Frank Sinatra, Bob Marley, and Eminem. Singing, jamming, rapping, and thinking.

What is this going to feel like?

Will I ever recover?

What if I don't wake up?

I dreamed all the things I was going to do after surgery that I had yet to do. For some reason, I never thought I was going to die. Not from this. Even through the pessimistic views, this wasn't my end. I don't know why. Maybe it was the calmness from the pain medicine or years of sports competitions "fight until the last buzzer." Regardless, I knew this was for the best, at that time in my life.

On surgery day, my parents, brother, and I prepped, joked, laughed, talked optimistically, and planned the fun we'd have post-surgery. Despite the chatter, nervous tension filled the room. That's when: "Mr. Godsey," and all present Godsey men answered, "Yes?" She laughed. "The patient. Brandon, I'm here to take you to surgery." Well, we all knew this was coming.

We proceeded into the elevator, down several floors into pre-op, and the doors to the next life opened. Nobody talked about it, but we all knew the scenarios. As the nurse started to wheel me in, I handed my iPod to my mom, opened to a playlist I created for her that was exactly the projected length of surgery, and cued to Bob Marley's "Every little thing, is gonna be alright."

As I let go of their hands, I said, "I love you guys. Thank you. See you soon."

The room was bright white with music blaring. I don't mean Frank. It was Nine Inch Nails. Heavy metal rock music at max volume. The nurse and I made eye contact, and she reassured me. "Don't worry. I know what you're thinking. I thought the same thing, but he's the best and he's in his zone. You're his third surgery today." If you think about it, as alarming as it was, I'd rather have him be in the zone with that, than out of the zone with Frank.

Anesthesia administered. Lights out.

CHAPTER 9: Post-Operation

06/29/2010:

Postoperatively, the patient was doing well.

On postoperative day #1, his IV fluids were decreased, advanced to a clear liquid diet, began to ambulate. He complained of significant pain and his PCA dose was increased. Otherwise the patient continued on postoperative day #3 on his PCA and clear liquid diet, had some nausea with clear liquid diet. His diet was continued to be advanced until he tolerated low residual diet on 07/02.

Instruction: *Patient was instructed to continue low fiber diet, not to lift anything heavier than a newspaper, walk around block. Patient was instructed to follow up with Dr. upon discharge and to return to the ER if he has a persistent fever, abdominal pain, intractable nausea or vomiting.*

90 minutes, 21 days, 40 pounds, and 1 fresh start.

Ninety minutes awoke in a sedated second's passing. My black lids lifted to the reality of living's adjusting. Consciously being brought three figures bedside. My mom softly leaned in. "Hi, sweetie." First movements smiled to lift from a lying position. The realization of the extent of surgery followed with an exuding discomfort throughout. Lying back to rest moved my insides around with a feeling that will nauseate me forever. Like water sloshing in a bucket, the freshly exposed and closed insides slid with exhaustive release. When you are cut open, pumped with air, cut out, and experience a surgery as severe, the aftermath will immobilize you while activating every pain receptor you possess. I set ten alarms on my phone to six-minute increments. Each ringing brought a half-squinted eye and a finger relieved to be pressing the trigger for a dose of self-injected Dilaudid.

Days passed and movements grew. Twenty-one total days in hospital Creme de la Creme was now left to grow one step at a time while staying as content as possible, gingerly propped on a bed to the most tolerable degree. An uncomfortable healing in the worst of ways. Forty pounds evaporated over the course of those days. Hair months past unkept. Body shrunken past the sickly "rail thin" to just bones. The smell of sickness stuck like days-old camp fire. Nevertheless, a week evolved from stretching to unguided bathroom staggers. Two weeks walked around the block. Weakness gained strength and Michigan gave peace to finish healing. Home for health. Home for the confusion. Home to start over. It took peeking at death to bring forth pure gratitude.

When you feel the wall behind you and the grave below, you're forced to fight. If you are lucky enough to survive the loaded gun of Russian roulette, take the time to understand all the whys of what you had to go through when you were where the how happened. Explore them all and be open to understanding what got you there. The remorse and confusion of surviving often distracts from progress toward finally stepping away from the disadvantageous path. This is a new start. Not a prolonged struggle. Walk and think and take every second you need to understand why you are still here and how everything you went through made you a better person for the life you get today. My strength grew not from my survival but from my family in that hospital and the talks that walked with health along that Lake Michigan shoreline. Routinely my mother and I strolled to those majestic summer sunsets, looking for sea glass and exploring life's conversations. Glass bottles that once attracted a purchase, was consumed by a soul a half century prior, tossed in the trash, legally thrown as waste into the lake, broken down for forty years, reformed, washed, pushed, polished, and reborn onto the shoreline as a symbol of survivor's beauty.

After a month, the question of what to do next finally became present. Persuasion played the hand of staying close to home, for precaution. The unfortunate thing for persuasion was that not for one moment had I ever thought of anything but finishing what I started in Los Angeles. Being an artist brought light into my confused life, and exploring its extremes had yet to commence. There was no doubt in my mind that I was going back to finish my training and to continue on. The problem was, in my twenty-five years, what had I done to change the habits that caused the madness? Minimal. Very minimal. Gluten and now fast food were gone. Well, most fast food. I knew other triggers, but half ignored them. You know, "I quit. Other than the 'occasional' In and Crohn's Out burger basket with fries and a shake. Because I'm doing better than the 'regular,' so it counts." You know, those justifications.

Regardless, I made it back. I continued on. I graduated that Meisner program, finished my improv training, and celebrated with beers and appetizer-smothered, covered, chunked, and drunk cheers. I was healed, but I hadn't learned my lesson. Time faded back into the "urgent rush," covering every grocery store bathroom in Southern California so routinely that I could tell you the location and restroom code before entering the store's sliding doors.

On production sets. On dates. On to the same ongoing onward disaster. On an island, held in an ignorant confusion. Fighting through the weakening imbalances. Friendships gained, friendships lost, isolation still had. Fun lived, careless exposed, life travelled. Reckless. So irresponsibly reckless in those years following. I may have gained relief from the pain, but I still had the disease. I told people I was changing and doing better. What I was, was walking again. Walking down the same road. The road to relapse.

On January 1, 2014, four and a half years after surgery, the clock struck midnight at a bougie burlesque club in Hollywood. Confetti's falling uncorked the bubbly and slowed the celebration to another near standstill. Like a dream, the lights dimmed to see a beautiful dress of cream and green eyes green. Love at first sight paused. That's when I met her. "You didn't think I was going to let you do this treatment alone, did you?" She wasn't new love, or exploring love. She was the feeling of healing one another from that moment forward love, and through our growing trust and commitment, the Changes would be set into motion.

04/24/14 MD Notes

Today, I saw Brandon Godsey in the UCLA Center for Inflammatory Bowel Disease in consultation. Brandon Godsey is a 29 y.o. male. The last 1.5 months his (Crohn's disease) symptoms have worsened. Patient reports colds, flus, lack of energy, poor mental stability, bad mood, diarrhea. Currently having 5 bowel movements a day. Soft, muddy, watery. Including 2 nocturnal bowel movements. Lower abdominal pain, cramping constant and also epigastric sharp squeezing pain. Subjective fever 2 days ago but did not check temperature. Right hip pain. No fissures/fistulas. Weight loss of 9 lbs/1 month. No appetite changes. Patient states that he would like to see someone for his depressed mood and anxiety because he is going through a "tough time."

Past Medical History:

- *Crohn's disease*
- *Anxiety*
- *Asthma*
- *Abscess*
- *Depression*

Workup will include the following:

-labs & stool
-colonoscopy with MAC for difficult sedation (pt had MAC previously) to assess extent and severity of disease, especially at anastomosis
-check MRE to rule out abscess, small bowel Crohn's
-f/u with PCP re: routine health maintenance (will refer to internal medicine)
-Patient interested in psychology/psychiatrist for mental health. Will encourage patient to follow up and schedule appointment with list of psychology/psychiatry providers
-Follow up in 6 weeks or sooner as needed

The house was again leaking with its weakening. My continuing lack of insurance, exhaustion, and justifications in a "healthy" fresh start, caused years of non-maintenance and untreated reasoning. Her persistence encouraged reestablishing a medical connection and pushed for progress. The insurance for all Obamacare fell in line with the timing. Finally, great insurance that restarted my ambition for not getting to the point I was before and scheduling an appointment with a "rising star" GI doctor at a local, well-regarded hospital. Regardless of the results or what developed next, love at first sight stepped in and started to correct the course.

05/02/14

TEST RESULTS:

Colonoscopy: Multiple scattered clean-based ulcerations noted throughout the visualized terminal ileum, extending more proximally beyond the scope, s/p biopsies. Post-surgical changes noted with widely patent ileocolonic anastomosis. There were a few small clean based ulcerations notes in the right colon at the area of the ileocolonic anastomosis which were biopsied. On retroflexion in the rectum, there was a large pedunculated polypoid mass at the dentate line, approximately 6cm in size, s/p biopsies. This was not removed given proximity to the dentate line.

Disease state:

Moderate disease activity

1. Symptomatic Crohn's disease, ileocolonic, currently on no medications with MRE 05/2014 showing 10cm thickening and enhancement of featureless TI with surrounding fat deposition and biopsies showing moderate chronic enteritis with erosion and granulomas

2. Depressed mood, likely related to Crohn's disease

3. Fatigue

4. Patient wishes to gain weight

Progress Notes:

Will plan for Remicade induction

The colonoscopy revealed activity around the area where the infected part of the intestine was cut out. The same area that showed healthy recovery after year one had developed the disease again by year four. Wearing my mind, body, and motivation into the bowels of the disease and left to fight, yet again. The colonoscopy also revealed a polyp at the end of the digestive tract, the rectum, that was not removed. Until obtaining my records for the book, we were always under the impression she removed the polyp, based on our post-colonoscopy consultation. Making the point of getting all the answers even stronger. Regardless, my condition was yet again fragile, and the next round of a different Crohn's-alleviating medicine was ordered.

"The only way to remission is to go on medicine. Remicade is a widely used drug that has had a lot of success. There is no cure to this disease and untreated will lead to another surgery. I recommend combining the Remicade and 6MP."

I declined the 6MP at the time, due to the stress one Crohn's medicine wears on the body and fear of not being able to handle multiple at once. Also, I had already experienced the discouraging course of 6MP in years past. Despite that small fact, it was still a pushed suggestion, and all I cared about was this chance at remission.

At that time, my emotions were either lusting in new love or away in depression. The disease was yet again touching all aspects of my life and causing confusion that channeled to my thoughts of living and were expressed with the angriest confused moments. Four years after learning my lesson, I had forgotten it. A year shy of five years and a year shy of the second surgery projection. Proving I hadn't learned a thing and medicine was agreed as being the most logical choice.

When it's all you know, how do you know anything else?

MD Notes:

Today, I saw Brandon Godsey in the Center for Inflammatory Bowel Disease for follow up visit. Now completed Remicade x3 infusions, with development of shingles 2 weeks ago. Last Remicade on 9/5/2014. Due for next Remicade on 10/30/14. Finished acyclovir per PCP on Monday x 10day course, ended last Wednesday. Positive for back pain and pruritis from skin lesions. Felt like Remicade worked for 2 weeks with more formed stools, energy, abdominal "relief," but reports having a constant cold with sinus issues, scratchy throat, fatigue, still abdominal cramping and now having 6 bowel movements a day, including 2 nocturnal and 1 this morning. With formed stools initially, then more watery urgent stools. Positive for shingles.

Current Outpatient Prescriptions Medication:
- fluticasone (FLONASE)
- hydrocodone-acetaminophen (NORCO)
- lidocaine-prilocaine (EMLA)
- lorazepam (ATIVAN)
- mirtazapine (REMERON)
- nortriptyline (PAMELOR)
- valacyclovir (VALTREX)
- VENTOLIN inhaler

Assessment & Plan:
1. Shingles outbreak
2. Immunocompromised state
3. Crohn's disease

Recommendations:

Patient instructed to follow up with PCP, re: shingles. Ok to delay 4th infusion of Remicade until shingles rash completely resolved (was due on 10/30/14 but will tentatively plan instead for 2 weeks later for ~11/13/14). Patient should extend acyclovir course if ok with PCP until next Remicade infusion. Labs today and with each Remicade infusion. Hold off on addition of 6-MP as combo therapy. Follow up within 4-6 weeks after Remicade infusion.

Crohn's disease took a back seat to my immunocompromised state, which was already in the back seat of a nasty shingles outbreak. All riding on the bus of relapse. Traveling down the road of solving one reaction's ailment with another prescription's writing. Three treatments it took to wear my body from bad to worse.

Shingles ensued, and so did months of painful exposure. What was I doing? Was this really how the story of my life was going to continually go? Would I stay with this approach and fight the disease while adding medicine to whatever else it wore me down to? The logic was missing, but I just couldn't figure it out. It wasn't clear yet. But what else was I going to do? Give in? Give up? Again, I'd never given up on anything in my life. I'd never failed at anything in my life. I'd be damned if I was going to just fade into the sunset of the disease and medicated sickness.

So, I went to the follow-up appointment. The shingles rash was down to a scar although the pain remained from toes to arm. The GI doctor was solely focused on getting back on track for treatments "progression."

What progression? Progression or regression? Then she said the last sentence I ever remember from her. "I knew you would probably get shingles. There's a good chance they will come back in the future. But we need to stay on the medicine. It's the only way for full remission."

It finally clicked.

And that was my 1 last treatment.

Chapter 10: The Solution

"This is a genetics-based disease. Unfortunately, there is no cure. It's tough to manage and even harder to put into remission."

Forget that. From this point forward, we've made the choice to get better, and because of that choice, we will. The odds may be next to nothing. Or impossible. Regardless, the choice is ours. Success germinates in the perception of accomplishment, and we can accomplish this. That's the only mindset. It's going to take time and commitment. There is no miracle pill.

Think back through my story. The day in college or youth to birth or the food habits and every single night in the hospital. How does that parallel with your course? What are you knowingly or unknowingly exposing yourself to? Let that honesty inform your new commitments with regard to food, lifestyle, and habits. Shift the trust from them (whomever they are) to you. *You.* You're going to build a new set of skills to survive our modern eating and lifestyle world. You can't be the best friend or sibling or spouse or parent, grandparent, teacher, and on and on, if you're not the best version of yourself.

Committing to the changes starts by forming new realistic spaces conducive to finally healing. A recovering alcoholic doesn't go into the same bar and expect to always order water. Instead they go to new places and spaces and build new sense memories around the habits they wish to have. If we are an alcoholic and stay in the presence of liquor, we'll always be tormented. Like going to a casino where tobacco is smoked and trying not to think about the cancer-causing habit you promised all your loved ones you'd quit. It's a little harder to hide when you're surrounded by the negative pleasure of temptation. Justification seizes opportunity in vulnerability. This new way of life— healing the gut and our living space of its toxic load—builds its foundation on the strength in new spaces.

PART I: Elimination

CHANGING THE LOGIC: Your Unique You

First commitment after walking out of those doors of your own "1 last treatment," or that old version of you, is finding a doctor or doctors who are open to all forms of healing and getting a full spectrum, blood food allergy test. Keep a copy of that test and all bloodwork for your personal records (along with all other transcripts) and take it with you to your appointments. File it, review it, and track your progress. What shows healthy today may be a deficiency tomorrow. Our bodies are exposed and developed in different ways, allergic to a completely unique set of substances. There'll be confirmed suspicions, surprises, and the never would've thought of, like thyme and safflower oil (a couple of mine). Unknown allergies hold us back. Find a way to get this test. For you. For the first step forward.

After the two months it took to heal the shingles, reality was finally out in front. If my body had worn down to the point of having a portion of its intestines removed, was wearing down again, and being given medicine that, in turn, was damaging my immune system to the point of exposing a disease that usually only reveals itself in the twilight years, what comes next? Something I probably can't come back from. One too many games of Russian roulette. This was my truth, and from that point forward I was forever committed, determined to figure

114

it out. No more blindly and unconsciously following the guided plan. No more doctors to "learn about this thing together" or "I knew it would come, but you need to stay on the medicine."

No more leaning. More standing tall.

The first place to start? The doctor. Without Dr. Maldonado, I may have gone untreated and a lingering abscess would probably have led to death. So, line up every doctor necessary and examine all possibilities to the fullest extent. Start with a primary care physician (PCP), or a functional medicine doctor, or a team lead like Dr. Maldonado. A confidant doctor, open to what you want and knowledgeable enough to make logical decisions based on current practices, proof, and methods.

After some research, I took the first step by joining my girlfriend to visit her chiropractor, who also practiced functional medicine. The twentieth-century's favorite alternative medicine labels—holistic and hippie—are now evolving into acceptance and continuing to grow in practice the more science and human knowledge expands. Western medicine sees a problem and provides a solution for that problem. Functional medicine focuses on restoring the body's balance by treating the entire body with a noninvasive approach: seeing the problem, finding the root causes, and using the body's own resources to build good health from an open understanding of diet, toxins, and lifestyle.

This doesn't mean throw away all medications tonight or give up on Western medicine tomorrow. It means expand your knowledge by exploring all routes. Find out what insurance will cover, and persistently fight to establish a wider range of experts and education.

Other ways of understanding the body. Other approaches. Other information. Other answers from everyone and everywhere you can. Let the collective results shape your decisions.

By the early spring of 2015, the car was in motion and we were on our way to the wellness doctor. Together, and finally committed to healing the battles. Tired of the agony and ready for the solution. She suffered from chronic back pain and endometriosis. Me, well, that's been well established. Although the appointment was originally for her, and we were to slip in the question of Crohn's disease, the conversation quickly changed to autoimmunity and the same solution for both of us.

"Wait, don't we have two completely different conditions?" I asked the doctor.

"It all starts with your gut and the restoring of balance. Hundreds of conditions are exposed because of an imbalance of one area." Okaay? What does that mean? "I'm going to order you a full spectrum blood food allergy test. We're going to eliminate what your body cannot process while implementing routines of natural substances and diet to heal while relieving the pressure."

"Ok, so I'm going on an assortment of pills? Isn't that the world I've spent a lifetime trapped in?"

"The difference is, chemical versus natural substances." Focusing on root causes while avoiding the damaging laundry list of side effects, like shingles. "Proper doses to balance the body and enhance operations for healing."

That logic, and what came from the rest of the appointment, turned out to be the best beginning I could've asked for. He showed what we would be testing and how it related to autoimmune diseases. We talked lab and price and went over the extent of his beliefs and why. He was honest, thorough, available, and open to ideas while confidently understanding how to heal without causing more harm. Just the kind of people we want to be surrounded by, especially our doctors. Coming from a place where asking my doctors for a simple dietician recommendation always made me feel small and frivolous, to being in a room with a person who understood, was open to discussion, available to the entirety of my past and current state, was not only refreshing but encouraging. Leaving that day, we felt confident the solution was real. The path was in front of us.

A week after blood was drawn, the results were in. Allergies to over fifty foods and substances that are commonly mixed into our everyday meals. Many favorites were finally exposed. Tomatoes, raw salmon, mushrooms. Apples, thyme, yeast. Knowing that false reports can happen, once my routine was in tune enough to incorporate and understand the effects of small amounts of each substance, I tested each and every one. Allergic to all was, and still is, confirmed. Maybe one day I will have restructured my cells to be able to tolerate them, but for now, it's not worth being fed grapes if they put me in hell.

CHANGING THE LOGIC: *Trust the Process*

Trust yourself, your results, and the process. Trust the food allergy test and remove the offending substances immediately, indefinitely. Cutting them from now until never is the only option. Check back with small amounts in a few years. Forget about it today. The fire will always stay lit when it has fuel, and we only have so much wood to burn. Allergies, toxins, stress, and inactivity all fuel the bonfire burning within.

117

As we walked out, pessimism was already analyzing the possibilities. The doctor's new regime was ten to fifteen supplements of powdered barks, natural ingredients, vitamin C, turmeric pills, a digestive enzyme, and fish oil, all while eating a "low residue" diet from a restricted food list of about twenty items. From a lifetime of endless food choices to a limited prison of twenty items and pills totaling nearly $200 for a four- to six-week supply. Realistic, not sustainable. Helpful, not quite the solution. "This seems very logical for healing, but we have to give up everything and can't eat anything! It's boring and bland! We can't be limited to only these foods? Plus, I'm a starving artist. I'll never be able to afford this." The justifications for failure were already accepted. A combination that was "extremely too difficult, but I'll give it a shot" was already the mindset.

A week in, we had held to form. Strict eating and taking all the pills on time. Then the truth of the situation showed up with our Sunday routine. Snacks, dips, booze, and a menu of "trying to do better" but too stubborn to give up the pleasures that go with the sense memories of our surroundings. We were not even close to understanding the changes we truly needed to make in every aspect of our lives for that doctor's method to come even remotely close to being possible. Beyond food there was stress; work; kitchen; pantry; bedroom items; household items; toxic loads that we breathe, ingest, and soak in; nutrition; molds; yeasts; infection; and so on. Lifetimes of habits that needed deprogramming. Lifetimes of being shaped into the present madness. The path may have been right there, but the solution was well down the road. Regardless, we were walking and optimistic.

This is what has happened to the gut over the progression of human history. We've been wearing down internally for generations. The Simple Change here is to empathize with that understanding while setting aside everything we've ever been taught through Western medicine. This is about scientific progression. We have advanced into a new understanding of the human body and are continuously moving faster, pioneering new solutions. So, it's time to drive out of the decades' old nutrition and lifestyle tunnel vision and welcome yourself into today's fast-paced and constantly expanding knowledge. Change is hard for all of us. Simple for science. In these times, embrace change by evolving with science.

There's the famous tale of Knute Rockne and his friend and player, George Gipp, the first All-American in Notre Dame football history. During the 1920 season George contracted strep throat and pneumonia from working on his craft after practice in the rain. Back then, there were no antibiotics. As he lay dying in his hospital bed, Rockne by his side, his last request for Rockne and the team was to "win just one for the Gipper." Rockne used those final words as inspiration for a half-time speech many years later, and Notre Dame came back to shock a highly ranked rival, Army, forever cementing the tale.

Two things stand out to me from that story. One, I would not have survived my strep throat during the Gipper times. Dead at age eleven. Antibiotics changed medicine while growing into the comfort solution (problem) it is now. Two, this is exactly why it's important we take care of ourselves now. The diseases that killed us back then, like polio, pneumonia, and colds, are nonexistent or easily treated now. The current diseases of the masses will be the most controlled ones later in our lifetime. We live longer now than we did then because medicine has advanced, and it's only speeding up, meaning we need to not only live healthily for today, but for the more days we will get to enjoy as our life expectancy expands. Autoimmune disease will be an easily treatable condition in our future. The near future. Right now.

Almost a fifth of the way through the twenty-first century, one in every six Americans suffers from one of over a hundred diagnosed autoimmune diseases. Another vast majority lives with developing symptoms. And the majority of the majority are women. All this adds up to nearly half the population of the United States, which is just one of many Western societies whose citizens suffer mild to severe stomach epidemics. Autoimmune disease went from a rare disorder in the 1980s to currently being the most common cause of death of individuals under the age of sixty-five. Autoimmune disease automatically qualifies us for being three times more likely to develop another, and the longer we live with it, the more severe it gets. This didn't come about by chance. We did this, humans and Adam Smith's evolution.

In order to push forward to solutions, we need to understand exactly what happens that makes us susceptible to becoming "autoimmune" in the first place. At conception we (usually) start with a perfect slate. Then somewhere along the line our growth is disrupted by an overload of antibiotics, steroids, stress, vaccinations, toxins, foods, and/or our modern "standard" practices. This causes bacteria to die and creates an imbalance in our body's microbiome—our healthy bacteria, viruses, fungi, and protozoa. These genetic materials exist everywhere on and in the body and are vital for fighting off invaders.

120

Now, zoom in on the gut, where everything consumed and absorbed breaks down and disperses throughout the body. It's also where 80 percent of the immune system resides. *Eighty percent* of this magical and mistakenly understood term "immune system" lives in the gut. The same place where bad bacteria can also live and flourish and cause disease. All bacteria, good and bad, fight continually and relentlessly for the same real estate.

With the gut wearing thin from toxic overload, the immune system senses an attack and goes into a defensive chaos. The irritation of imbalances forces the healthy army to blindly fight back. The immune system is confused and starts attacking its own tissue and cells, healthy or not. It is the same principle as how antibiotics work: no differentiation, just demolition to get rid of all bad, regardless of the good in the way. From here, tight junctions between cell walls loosen, unwarranted bacteria and organ connections establish, inflammation tries to evoke healing, and the damaged area enlarges with our continued poor food and lifestyle habits. The result? The immune system becomes an unknowing ally of the damaging condition that has already invaded and begun to establish within the gut.

This swelling throughout the tract—inflammation—makes it even more difficult for food to be absorbed, harden, and healthily move into waste as it passes through. Normally, the small spaces in cell walls allow only tiny healthy macronutrients to travel from the breaking-down food into the bloodstream and from there to organs and operating processes throughout the body. Like Oompa Loompas marching to their happy (and slightly creepy) tune as they carry materials throughout the mini-size functional, large-person-size factory. Now picture the toxic overload opening the doors wide for all those ungrateful kids to enjoy. Microbes, toxins, proteins, and partially digested large particles of food now running free in the bloodstream, falling face first into the chocolate river. This is what is known as a "leaky gut."

Leaky gut is just one of the many effects a depleted microbiome and compromised immune system develop into. Leaky gut loosens stools, deprives the body of nutrients, and carries bad bacteria and infections into other parts of the body, and that can develop into highly inflammatory and chronic conditions like Crohn's disease or an abscess on the liver or arthritis, asthma, endometriosis, and hundreds of associated conditions. Chronic inflammatory conditions that can then develop into cancers and other conditions we can't come back from.

From here, the immune system and gut wear to a point of no return—autoimmunity—and, as nearly every professional over several decades has said, once you become autoimmune "there is no current cure."

Stating there is not a cure is misleading and makes us believe we are stuck with our conditions forever. The cure is remission by creating new habits and spaces.

Autoimmunity correlates to our cultural shift of becoming afraid of bacteria. Or as Doctor For-Life would put it, "the cleanliness disease," a phrase I once naively thought meant showering and washing my hands too much. Although that is part of it.

Our bodies are no longer exposed to certain pathogens they were exposed to generations ago. Industrialized nations have cleaned them away with antibiotics, sanitizers, cleaning chemicals, water treatment, manufacturing, and food processing. Western societies have a third less bacteria on average than undeveloped nations. This means that our personal society—our body—is now trying to protect itself with a third fewer healthy occupants. And the enemy—infections, yeasts, fungus, disease—is always waiting and evolving. Enter the quick fix: system obeying, fear instilling, flu shots, vaccines, and any other preventatives.

CHANGING THE LOGIC: *Healing the Home*

Remain thoughtful of what is being changed and what needs to be changed. Start with the basics: home and its food, products, and everyday exposure to toxins. Get used to understanding product labels by dissecting what's on the back and ignoring the manipulative, cleverly marketed for your subconscious appeal, front. Replace the products in your home to lessen your toxic exposure and throw away all food you're consciously, or unconsciously, poisoning your body with. We spend 50 to 70 percent of our lives at home. That means you live over half of the Simple Changes in one space.

My Digestion-Activating Stretches Suggestions: There's nothing like waking from a good night's dream that refreshingly moves into a long morning stretch. Before rising, move through a set of digestion-activating, abdominal-releasing stretches and twists. Hug knees to the chest for thirty seconds. Drop your left arm, palm up, to the left. Right arm cradles the knees that drop to the right. Hold for thirty seconds. Knees back to the chest. Hold. And reverse. Morning-stretch it out one time. Now, feet to a butterfly position and pelvis in the air. Thirty seconds with arms overhead. Knees to the chest. Breathe. Now, everybody clap your hands. Cha cha real smooth.

Stretching can seem daunting until we think of it as something else, like incorporating DJ Casper into the mix. Add in a couple more twists to the morning, brush those toxins out, and let's roll over into the kitchen.

My Morning Water Tips: Stove on, purified water in, heat up, slight boil, and drink. Or, later on in the healing, add fresh herbs to an unbleached tea bag, squeeze the lemon, sprinkle the cinnamon, and steep for three to five minutes. Consume 20 to 30 minutes before a meal. The body has gone six to eight hours without any food or water; this gives it time to rehydrate before the work begins again. Grab your doctor-assisted, plan-laid-out dose of supplements. Mine at this time were vitamin C, a turmeric pill, a digestive enzyme pill. Wash them down, again, 20 to 30 minutes before a meal to allow them time to dissolve. Enjoy that calming nourishing tea with a few deep breaths, and welcome to the first day of understanding the changes.

Sipping and prepping. Washing and chopping. Grabbing the eco-friendly nontoxic ceramic skillet, flipping the heat to medium, and sprinkling in unrefined extra-virgin olive oil. A healthy anti-inflammatory oil to boost the immune system while promoting healthy cell repair and growth, used here to sauté a sweet potato hash. Once browned, push it to the pan's side and fill the space with a couple multicolored, locally sourced, organic, no corn or soy fed, chicken eggs from a friend with an honest reputation. Cook the organic turkey bacon, fix the organic tomatillo salsa, organic refried pinto beans, organic homemade guac, finish with organic corn tortillas, top with nonrennet goat cheese, and breakfast has been deliciously healthified. Numerous common toxins and artificial ingredients like pesticides, low quality immune system–suppressing oils, and known

124

allergens have already been removed from your day. A meal that avoids the bad while providing the body with good.

(A note on organic foods: They used to be more expensive than nonorganic foods, but that has changed, and it's now perfectly possible to source organic products that are priced the same as nonorganic. Shop around. Also, if you need to, check the Environmental Working Group's [EWG] Clean 15 list for nonorganic produce that is least contaminated with harmful pesticides.)

Pour the champagne for the significant other and fix a specialty Moscow mule for the gentleman. "Ahhh, Sunday morning."

That may have sounded perfectly healthy. But I was still holding on to the goat cheese, eggs, and bacon, and I was still exposing myself to detrimental food combinations (like grains and nightshades) that I didn't yet know about. Also, the expense of that meal wasn't efficient. Quality is the one thing that cannot be sacrificed in the healing process, and those dozen eggs cost three times the price of the lowest quality eggs. However, eggs are not even a part of the final healing solution. There are enough affordable combinations of foods that will heal you.

On this, your first day of changes, it's not what's eaten but what's absorbed, both internally and informationally. Some foods take three days to show an allergic reaction, and one trace of a damaging substance—gluten, for example—can take three months to remove and heal from. Sadly, cross contamination can happen through a food being processed either with the same machine or using a similar practice that blends our good with our banned substances. To that, goodbye all dairy, all gluten, everything on your allergen food list, and granulated sugars. Goodbye chemical-laden low-quality pans. Adios highly processed and low-quality oils. Hello unrefined extra-virgin organic olive oil or unprocessed (virgin) organic coconut or avocado oil. These may be a little more expensive but are used in small quantities and take longer to use up. Our first cocktail mixers of that day, like sweet and sour, gets transformed into this day's fresh lime juice, ginger juice, organic potato vodka, and muddled mint, shaken and poured into a classically refreshing copper mug. Just like getting the medical care that you deserve, you can't skip these changes. You have to find a way to make it work for you. For products I have used to heal myself, take a look at my website www.MySimpleChanges.com/products. In fact, if there's ever any part of the changes you'd like extra help with, the website connects you with videos, brands, professionals, and more of what I wish I'd had during my healing.

My Portions Tips: Before serving, shift your awareness to the dangers of overeating. The change here is smaller, more frequent, highest quality, meals. Make your normal portion and before even taking that first incredible bite, put half into a glass storage container and leave it for later. After taking the first bite, pause before the next. Slower consumption of a smaller meal allows digestion to operate more efficiently, easing stress on the system while the healing substances are better absorbed (like turmeric. ginger, and bone broth...explained more on page 202).

"I get the less consumption. But why glass? My plastic is BPA free!"

The goal is to eliminate all known and/or potential toxins with the most assured, highest quality products and ingredients. Therefore, wherever beliefs fall or comprehension stands, when it comes to plastic, it's best to avoid every form and go with the proven toxin-free option. For the fridge, the pantry, the cabinets, the spices and herbs, the to-go, the storage, and everything else that falls into your version of the My Simple Changes routine. For you, for removing exposure, for portion control, for healthy leftovers, for the plastic-polluted environment, for our future restored self, and for our children.

"Glass is too expensive. I got my plastic take-out. AKA free!"

Glass is an investment that holds up as long as time. No more justifying. Change and move forward before the plastic breaks down, leaches, and continues to increase your toxic load.

With half of the hash stored, "Breakfast is prepared, my love." The romantic in me loves to spoil her, like it should be, and set up brunch on a small table in the sand between our beach chairs and the bay. We learn from whom we grow with. Food, lifestyle, and dating. Thankfully, chivalry was developed by understanding my father's suave ways of what not to do, like that first date of homemade wine and nibbled cheese. Cheers. "To Grandpa McCoy's wine, our love, and growing health."

Breakfast by the bay. Just as good as Mom's apple pancakes on vacation. The greatest memories of growing up, my friends and family pouring that warm, high-fructose corn syrup ("maple syrup") onto those fresh, fluffy apple pancakes. The same love, same time shared, and same appreciation of location. Same emotions, different foods, same taste memory fulfillment. Proving it's not the food but the company that creates the moment.

Our idyll was disrupted by the howling sound of a nearby ship's midday horn. One more deep breath, taking in the surrounding senses. Our hands unlocked and the rest of the day called for attention. Breakfast's conversation would become a Sunday boardwalk bike ride to our spot, but first the cleaning, the chores, the getting ready. The efficiency of maintaining a clean and organized home while preparing for the next adventure.

Sort the load of laundry, scrub the mound of dishes, and vacuum the inevitable collection away. The counters wiped with a cost-efficient organic cotton towel, and not with the inhalation of normal disinfecting toxins but with the increased efficiency of a homemade vinegar and lemon combination. A HEPA air filter ventilated the open windows' passing of a cool Pacific Ocean breeze. Between toxin-eliminating plants, open air, and the HEPA filter, toxins were eaten away and spit out fresh, ready for our lungs to heal with every inhale and cleanly exhaust with every release.

With the chores done, it was now time for a quick shower.

My Showering Suggestion: Get in, get busy, sing one song, get out, and don't come again for a few days, to keep the oils, bacteria, and naturals alive and well throughout the entire microbiome (in this case, skin, hair, and inhalations of steam). Conscious of not getting too clean through the use of chemicals, I switched shampoos, body washes, and conditioners for essential oil or plant-based organic ingredients. Going for a GOTS-certified organic towel, nontoxic hand soap, and brushing with a bamboo toothbrush and toothpaste that avoids fluoride, minimizes ingredients, and is natural, eco-friendly, and plant based.

Deodorants, lotions, and hair health are all happily replaced with high-quality essential oils and homemade products. Essential oil deodorant of peppermint, lavender, and tea tree mixed in a glass spray bottle and diluted with purified water now sprays under each arm and coats with a natural coconut oil sealing blend. Essential oil lotions formulate around individualized ailments and are blended with a carrier oil like unrefined organic coconut oil, extra-virgin olive oil, or shea butter, all great for rehydrating and repairing skin cells.

To the mirror's reveal, hands rub any residue into receding locks of increasingly distinguished gray. Another gene passed from my father, father's father, and generations before. This one, I can't change other than to soothe the follicles while reviving natural oils and cleaning the roots by removing toxins.

Fresh laundry, washed with nontoxic unscented soap and chemical-free dryer balls and warmly covering a happy chihuahua who burrows in.

Again, to help lighten the daunting load, all products and helpful tools can be found on the www.MySimpleChanges.com website.

Many common staple products have grown into oversaturated, low-quality options. Making better choices as to what you use in your home and on your body reduces the harmful chemicals that can be absorbed into your system and subsequently block communication between cells.

My Toxins Tip: As silly as each of my explained changes may seem, removing one toxin at a time over the course of time, is the solution. It's not one toxin, it's all of them combined that make up our toxic load that exposes autoimmunity.

In the same way, foods that were once perceived as healthy, and justified with phrases such as "my grandparents ate it and they were fine," are now victims of science, cost efficiency, and the hybridization of foods. Genetically integrating two strains of wheat to make a new strain allowed wheat to become water soluble and in turn used as a thickener that expanded its use beyond bread. That doesn't mean we possess the necessary pathogens to digest it. The truth now is, bread is nothing naturally close to what your grandparents used to eat, and we are now exposed to scientifically engineered gluten in countless ways other than just food, for example medications, beauty products, and more.

"Yeah, that's why I buy gluten-free bread! So, I'm already doing better!"

Not quite. Gluten-free can mean, if the product is low quality, that the gluten is replaced by chemically laced sugar, gut-irritating acids, and processed flours. Gluten is just one example in a food industry affected throughout by the same evolution. Remove from the experiment. Become the observer by making the right changes. Whole foods, prepared and broken down by you.

CHANGING THE LOGIC: How to Survive Eating at Restaurants

Before even deciding on the place, search for restaurants that serve fresh, organic food and/or list all the ingredients on their menu. We want places that take pride in the quality of the food they serve, not the lowest quality great taste they can get away with. If you're not in on the establishment decision, look up the menu beforehand and know exactly what and how you are going to order. Going in blind is justification's eventual poor decision. A solid strategy is the Simple Change. Even go to the extent of calling the restaurant and asking your way through a plan around your restrictions. No more being shy about the imperfectly perfect requirements of your body. From there, choose individual whole-ingredient dishes without sauces, spices, and low-quality oils or butter. Let you be the one to put on the citrus, oil, and herbs. "Spices" could mean anything, including thyme or cilantro or something you're allergic to. And, if, just if, you can't avoid exposure to what you've nixed, eat beforehand and just order a small salad or steamed veggies that fall under the EWG.org Clean 15.

"After you, madam."

We set the pedals in motion and, like a scene from *Groundhog Day*, the boardwalk's bush got the best of her again. Connected and crashed for the third time this month. Motor skills, B+. Balancing a bicycle in narrow spaces, C-. Lifting her up, we were off, again. First break, exactly one roadie's length in the California sun to a bottomless patio party. Bottomless mimosas, that is, executing the "cancel ride" to perfection. "Alcohol plus exercise removes toxicity," said Johnny Justification.

Drinks later: "My drink found bottom." Answering her call: "My stomach found empty." Perking up: "Mexican cantina?"

That was our spot! That place with a great bar and even better bartender. Where drinks muddle from scratch and authentically concoct to the perfection of your liking. Where your pickiness for particulars are understood. A place like this, the bartender knows your needs and captures a My Simple Changes perfect margarita to professional perfection. Floated drinks and salted rims sided two baskets of chips that backed up to a three-dip pairing of refried beans, salsa, and guac. Upward glances settled to tuning in and smiles embraced the world that remained tuned out. Glasses raised for surviving the ride, well, sort of. "To a great, healthy day and doing exactly what we love to share together. Drinking, eating, and being. Cheers, babe!"

One drink later found intoxicated boasting. "I can look at a dish or menu and highlight toxic exposures of each ingredient. That's what my obsession has grown into! Almost as if words with arrows highlight each damaging scenario." A true statement, as odd as it seems. From seed to consumption, my degree in logistics has been put to good use by understanding the flaws imposed by the process. A decade in the service industry proved to be perfect training for this relentless pursuit through years of meals and linking answers through paying attention and self-education. Now transformed into analyzing all circumstances while piecing together the best solution.

Here's the problem with our average restaurants and the fast food places that control our college hangovers and drug-induced decisions. Food cooked, frozen, reheated, and refreshed in sauces is not real food. Moving a step backward, the same food delivered by a "service" specializing in moving bulk frozen foods to the aforementioned restaurants and fast food places comes from independent contracts with companies specializing in decreasing bottom lines by improving shelf life with enhanced preservation of taste and texture. This is not a new concept. In fact, its decades old. Same mindset, much larger scale. Same mindset, more lab-created substances. Same mindset, and let's take one step farther back.

Super seeds. Seeds scientifically changed to withstand Mother Nature's all, while growing fruitfully colorful and tall. The genetically altered food rabbit hole soaking into toxin-compromised soil. From seed to consumption, each layer in the supply chain process is altered with methods that pay no attention to our gut's abilities. Super seeds, "natural flavors" prepared with preservatives during processing, freezer ready, boxed, stored, shipped, stored, ordered, microwaved, fried, mixed with other seasonings and ingredients of the same assemblages, or shelved with the creative genius of analytics-based cleverly created characters, colors, and words. Like going into a donut shop as a kid and seeing a smiling bunny holding a plastic bottle of chocolate milk and bright words promoting "great for calcium!" and the engrained mindset of "dunk that donut!" At the other end of the chain, our gut is subjected to the infinite exposures that our modern systematic food processes create.

Meats, apart from what our "modern methods" have done to our greenhouse gas problems, follow the same path to the table.

Controlled by scientific advancement that's driven from the concept of furthering economic growth while controlling costs and producing more. The evolution of man and food. It started well before our understanding. Decades of decisions from unrelated trades, tariffs, regulations, and union costs forced the United States economy into becoming a service industry in the late 1970s. Foods were outsourced to unregulated lands, and parts were made in Mexico, assembled in Thailand, packaged in Central America, and sent through the supply chain of an American company, resulting in lower costs, lower quality, and the loss of industry and jobs in little cities like Buchanan, Michigan. Industries in small towns were forced to change their methods in order to meet margins. For example, bringing in fish that's caught off the toxic coast of wherever, sent frozen by boat for processing in Thailand, and shipped here in the same way to sit on shelves or freezers in preserving solutions awaiting our consumer decisions.

"What happens when we're at the airport, on a bus, in a hotel room, on holiday travels, hiking, camping, infinity, and beyond?"

The same as the restaurant: Plan a strategy to the best of your ability and as far in advance as realistically possible. Bring food, eat beforehand, prepare, research, evaluate options, and consume conscious amounts of purified water. Just as with identifying the ingredients of "Sunday Funday's" restaurant menu, the more you grow into the changes, the easier the solutions come together. It seems impossible, until it shows possible. Patience, time, and persistence.

CHANGING THE LOGIC: Sleep

Sleep. First, avoid eating a couple of hours before bed. Next, before fading into mimi's, end the day how it started with warm water, stretches, and an unwinding stillness. Feel deep breaths and appreciate the bed we get to lie in ready for another peaceful slumber. Six to eight hours of sleep isn't an old wives' tale. It's an old tale holding up through time and becoming scientifically proven. The body may go into rest mode while being under the spell, but this is a twenty-four-hour shop, and repair takes place during the different levels of inactivity. Those levels need to be as undisturbed as possible for the optimal healing we're devoting a third of our life to. We already cut out gluten and dairy. Getting an extra hour or two of sleep is a Simple Change that will lower inflammation, help stabilize C-reactive protein levels, and ultimately aid in repairing and recharging the body properly for another day. Don't sleep on cutting sleep. Prioritize it with the most nontoxic bedroom possible.

We rode home to a cold chill that pushed along a path illuminated only by our flashing reflectors and the distant lights of a bay filled with container ships. To the flows of Chris Stapleton and the waves crashing in the darkness, away from the world we stayed present in the great day's final moments. Happiness and exercise, just as important as toxins and food.

By the time we got home, extreme thirst sobered our arrival. Not drinking water or fluids during a meal is another Simple Change. Drinking during meals dilutes our natural stomach acids and disrupts the breaking down of food. Forgetting to drink water throughout the day? Dries up the machine. Find the balance. Which reminds me, how much water was consumed during this one day? How much water of every day contaminates the microbiome and gut environment? How much of the day's water is purified, free of toxins and fluoride? How much did we forget to sip throughout the day?

My Daily Water Consumption Strategy: The Simple Change aims for at least a liter and a half (64 to 100 ounces a day), while identifying and limiting exposure to toxin-bearing water. Added minerals and substances like fluoride are easily removed by being aware and replacing with reverse-osmosis, alkaline, and purified water stored in glass, through filters, or refilling a nontoxic bottle at the store purifying machine for .35 cents a gallon. Make this one change and easily reduce the toxic buildup by cleaning, flushing, lubricating, and hydrating.

Think of the water through this one day. Tea or hot water, followed by ice cubes for drinks, washing food and dishes, showering (skin and inhalation), brushing teeth, restaurant lemon water, washing hands, homemade cleaners and deodorant, laundry, before-bed warm water, and the diffuser. Common scenarios we're exposed to on a daily basis.

Our water has been heavily exposed to toxins deep within the ground, in the oceans, and in treatment within each city. Industrialization, narrow-minded practices, and the rabbit hole of evolution have created an environment where it isn't as easy to consume pure water. For instance, the former Electro-Voice facility that once contributed to powering my childhood hometown was forced to leave because of their unregulated discharging of electroplating wastes into two of our city's lagoons, contaminating the groundwater with chemicals called volatile organic compounds, or VOCs (become accustomed to understanding exposure to those). The EPA forced a cleanup and Electro-Voice found a new home for offices and production in another state and country. That's just one of countless examples of damage caused in loosely regulated industrialized nations, making the need to stay informed today, and every day moving forward, that much more crucial.

While enjoying a movie, book, project, or something to further the imagination and happy your ways, stretch. Breathe. Relax. Take time to appreciate what today gave before closing it and getting back at it tomorrow. Call that person. Check in to the mind's eye. Turn on the diffuser blended with the best relaxing essential oils like lavender, eucalyptus, and frankincense. Or sip some hot tea while breathing deep into the aroma. Drink some of that purified water before bed, cuddle into the peace of those 100 percent EOS-certified organic cotton sheets, and get those six to eight hours of sleep the body needs for repairing, refueling, and regrouping. Stretch for digestion, listen to the calm, share one last appreciation, and fade into the happy rest of getting to build it all again tomorrow.

PART II: Stress

You can take life in two ways. The way it affects you or the other way: the way it is. Leave the world of being affected, by enlisting in your new space. Ralph Waldo Emerson once wrote, "A man is what he thinks about all day long." The truth of what is, is that we are all going through it and we are all being held down in some way by it. The more we can be open to understanding that, the less time we'll spend in the space of being affected by it. Unfortunately, the curve to understanding comes though progression of resolving. The quicker we understand the resolve, the healthier and more available our body will be to build.

Which brings us to one of the biggest criminals in life. What is it? One that wears us of our every day potential? Oh, you know what this is. It's that thing in the gut, the chest, the breath, the legs, the mind, and the heart. It's carried with us. Shapes our mood and sentences. Heightens anxiety. Causes sadness, depression, lack of motivation and focus. It dictates digestion. Speeds up our walk. Shallows our breaths. Churns our stomach. Shortens our lives. The constant feeling of hurt in our torso, that wears to tears and exposes the most vulnerable parts within. It's different for everyone but felt the same by all.

Stress.

CHANGING THE LOGIC: *Identifying and Removing Peer Pressure*

Understand which peers are pressuring you and how you can keep the right distance without giving in to their standards. Find that balance of them and the changes you now live and breathe. Your standards will never again be the same as anyone else's. The change is finally standing up for your standards, while politely declining theirs.

"I'm just going to make some tacos and have a kombucha," I said to her in response to supper's fixing.

"You're not going to have any of Papa's chicken or the dinner we made for you?" Even though she already knew I couldn't.

"No, thank you. I want to, but I'm allergic to the tomatoes and shouldn't be eating the chicken."

Replying with her fingers two inches apart from one another: "Oh come on. I only put in *this* much tomato! Do you *really* think that much is going to affect you?"

Guilt mounting. "I really shouldn't. I don't want to ruin progress. I've been feeling better."

"I read all chicken is the same anyways. Organic or not."

"It's more than that."

They all look on with a skeptical hurt as the mother, again, puts her fingers up to show how much tomato sauce was in the dish. "Come on, Brandon." Three against one. Justification's campaign committee of peer pressure persuasion.

"I guess it won't hurt." I gave in, solely to appease and silence. Don't get me wrong, the food was delicious. But the decision was detrimental and the effects were the same.

The next morning sluggishly came and I dragged my way to a callback audition for a commercial. The kind of gig that makes the artist's survival meter go from flashing red to relief's green. After LA traffic's dangers, the meal tossed its churn and a full rush hit for release. Last night's dinner was now showing its denial—or damaging exit, I should say—all hitting to the timing of a casting assistant's calling, "Brandon Godsey." No time for the bathroom now. I was sweating and holding in rush-like contractions, just like in that scissor lift during practice with nowhere to go. I walked in the room, mind occupied by the angry grips that is Crohn's disease, distracted from any thought of the great opportunity at hand. Audition focus and clarity opened the door, and failure of my personal responsibility shut it. My defeated exit wedged through the crowd of actors waiting to fill one role, and a hallway's walk-turned-sprint found the bathroom.

That food may have tasted delicioso, but the harmful results remained in the smell of the toxins' infectious waste. Allergy-flaring ingredients plagued the bathroom atmosphere. A stomach, its vital acids and bile, undigested tomatoes, and hidden toxins triggered the bad bacteria waterslide, and all jumped on at once. Reset button pushed. Months of hard work now back to square one. When all of a sudden, *creeeeeak*. The door opened, and a man entered the stall next to me. I held to only a subtle eye movement, embarrassed. His sheer repulsion exclaimed, "Oh my god!"

Wait, a second. That's not a man.

"That's horrible!"

With a dropping heart and frantic eyes, I looked around to see some smell-good flowers and a disposable waste box.

"You were?" my friend asked while at drinks that evening.

"Yep."

No urinal. Sheer embarrassment. Audition fail, bathroom-relief fail, and still captive in the ten-second pleasure followed by days-of-pain fail.

"Why did you eat that food?"

"They bullied me! What else was I going to do?"

The one skeptic at the table asked, "Isn't Crohn's disease genetic?"

This isn't an unusual conversation. Actually, it's more routine than one would believe. "I shouldn't even be drinking this vodka right now, really. But I do to be here with you guys, so." The truth of it all.

"Food doesn't cause it, man," someone else said.

"Here we go again." My chipper reply from years of repetitive conversations.

"Oh, leave Brandon alone. He's our sensitive friend, remember?"

Tired of being around people insensitive to my conditions, I said, "You know what, I think I'm going to go. It's been a long, women's room defeating kind of day."

The congenial friend of the group tried to ease the tension. "Oh come on, man, we never get to hang out anymore and I just ordered tomato soup for the table!"

"No thanks, man. Eat it for breakfast. I'll see you guys next time."

Walking out as whispering conversation faded through the window, I heard, "It's really hard going anywhere with him. He has so many allergies!" "Does he really think he can cure it?" "He just melts like a snowflake! What a baby. He should just go back on the medicine."

Days like this fill a disease.

This is the truth a person living with illness hears throughout their "different than normal" lives. Whatever normal is anymore. I missed a lot of my life and valuable moments by being sick. Moments I wanted. Moments I would've loved to share. I flaked on so many people and cancelled so many auditions and jobs. Nobody has time for flakes, this is true. But flakes usually go do something more appealing, not lie in bed for days, depressed, exhausted, and lost in what they're living with. No matter how much I would explain, it never seemed to change the thoughts people held around me. It's much easier to prove a broken arm than an inside that feels like an army of diseased zombies are dancing in spiked shoes to Michael Jackson's "Thriller."

That was my elephant in the room. Suffering through the disease and suffering through stress and being controlled by the different levels it takes us to. We know it keeps us from the full extent of our happiness, yet few of us recognize how to get rid of it. We don't take the time to identify the depths to which it closes us off, tightens us, and ultimately exposes us to worsening health conditions. Stress channels through over (or under) eating, substance abuse, social withdrawal, or wiping our energy to inactive slumber. No two people are the same, and the root causes combine in a different way for each and every one of us. Job, health, family, friends, illness, death, breakups, money, loneliness, and the material things in life that we care so much about but are not even real in the first place. We can't touch stress. We can only feel it.

From well before I was diagnosed with Crohn's disease until years after surgery, I lived with stress. Trapped in life's darkest shadows. The shadows that allow you to be you during the day while anxiously waiting to run away with you at night. Or the ones that keep you away during the day, forcing you to regret your life at night. You know, the places we're not proud of but "the Crohn's is gonna get me in the end anyways." So, who cares? "Pass the special, special. Cheers!"

With that controlling logic there's no need to even think beyond the detrimental short-term relief. Self-destruction to the point of being held together by only the thread of the few who love us the most.

CHANGING THE LOGIC: Channeling Life's Inevitable

At age nine, fifty-eight, twenty-five, 103, whenever, eventually life forces us to question our existence and sends us on a search to find inner peace. In a time where it's easier to give up and succumb to justifications, take the opportunity and build the loss into growth. Reshape the space to include healing routines, ones that work with the body's natural processes to calm during a difficult time. The inevitable is a fact, and in a moment's notice it will come. What you can control is how to channel it before it channels you and leads you down the rabbit hole of autoimmunity.

In May of 2016, I was carrying groceries inside and missed a call from my grandmother. They were now in an assisted living home in Michigan, where my dad and mom could take care of them. She was happy despite the circumstances. By this time Grandpa had left parts of himself in the past. Dementia constantly challenged his everyday situation. "Brandon. This is Grandma. I'm sorry I missed your call earlier. I was getting my hair done. I'll try again later. Take care now. Bye-bye, honey."

Two nights later, she passed in her sleep.

A great friend to so many. A major piece in our support system left in the middle of the night. Her death had a large effect on me. Missing her last call hurt. Now I cherish the voicemail. That's all we have left. The voicemails, most sacred items, and mementos from their sixty-four-year love story together. The stretched truth that I told her in our talks were the same ones I used to convince the rest of the world I was doing ok. All to avoid the perception of doubt or words that added to the hurt within. She knew. She was a smart and attentive woman.

Unfortunately, those lies of health and happiness justify their way into our everyday. We all feel the age where our own mortality starts to truly sink in. This life event finally brought my emotional health into focus. The dark spaces of my life, the progress of already made changes, and her lasting impression combined to set off a chain reaction to finally solving the pain that I had carried for far too long. In order to heal the gut, I need to address the stress.

Stress centers around the central nervous system, which relays all of the messages from the brain through the limbs, organs, gut, and throughout. Hundreds and hundreds of millions of nerves

144

communicating how each and every part is doing, feeling, and working. When acute stress responses happen (more commonly known as "fight or flight"), cortisol and adrenaline release from the brain into the body and the digestive system gets thrown into chaos. Everything tightens and the central nervous system cuts off blood flow, disrupting the normal contractions of digestive muscles.

In the first half of the stomach, where food starts to break apart, a stress reaction causes the process to shut down, which results in severe nausea and extended discomfort. Stress then works its way down into the gastrointestinal tract and prompts intestinal spasms, either forcing the system to flush out or back up, which then triggers an intestinal flare-up and prevents nutrients from being appropriately absorbed. Stress and gut health are not a case of one causing the other. They feed off one another to worsen the condition.

So, how do you heal from *your* stress and aid in healing the gut?

YOGA

While asking for a referral to a dietician and talking about curcumin supplements as an "alternative option that may help slightly relieve symptoms," I asked my GI doctor if he recommended yoga. "It won't cure you but may help with the stress," was his auto-response. He also said nothing was going to heal me besides the medicine. So, I didn't really take yoga into serious consideration. From that moment until finally going to a class, I thought about it a million times and always justified a way out, mainly for the same reasons we all avoid taking the leap into anything new. We fear change, trust, and perception. Frankly, it wasn't "manly" for men to do yoga. Or at least that's the impression my "manly" friends gave me.

When I first started practicing, one stretch in particular became my gauge for improvement: a reverse bridge pose. Lying on my back, knees bent and feet on the ground, lifting the hips in the air while tucking my shoulder blades down and as close as possible under my back. Mixing that with a combination of twists and deep breathing. Over time the throbbing pain in the Crohn's-infected area of my intestine calmed to a dull ache and has now evolved into nothing but a normal stretch.

Relaxing into a breath while holding a pose allows the body to speak. Shallow breathing is a direct result of stress and tightens the body's process, which causes further stress. Yoga challenges us to open and deepen focused breath, eventually allowing us to release what we've been holding in and shallowly breathing through for so long. Picture those goofy poses you could never embarrassingly get yourself to do because everyone else would see you. Wrong. Yoga is for all shapes, sizes, and flexibility, and if you're practicing yoga, you don't see anyone else seeing you, because you are so focused you don't have time to care about another's judgment. In through the nose, out through the mouth. Deep breaths. Not only does relief come from the relaxation, yoga offers a free gauge of how much the body is healing and strengthening over time.

Breath, flexibility, and, most importantly, aid in regulating digestion. The deep stretching, different twists, and focused poses help by draining the lymph nodes of toxins, increasing blood flow, building muscle strength, improving posture, and supporting the regulation of adrenal glands. All of which play a part in healing inflammation, the immune system, the digestive tract, stress, and ultimately symptoms from ailments and/or diseases.

This may seem frivolous and unbelievable. But a one-solution mind lacks the vision to connect the changes and understand the patience of time's healing. Yoga works, but only if it's worked into your routine and you trust it's working.

You can find suggested yoga videos at https://mysimplechanges.com/collections/exercise. Or find a class with an instructor who makes you feel welcome and encourages you to attend more often.

My Yoga Routine: I aim for practicing yoga at least two times a week, with a goal of four. Remember, it's a practice. Not a perfect. And there is no practice, unless you're there.

MEDITATION

"I'm getting more sleep, changing my food, exercising, I am making the changes!"

Close, but not quite. This is a forever evolution of change, and the next step out of the comfort zone is meditation. Understanding the power of meditation can only be achieved by routinely committing to it, taking yourself to a quiet place, getting comfortable, and focusing on each breath with localized scans of the body, all while releasing thoughts and increasing blood flow to inflamed areas.

My Meditation Routine: Twice a day. Ten-minute sessions, at minimum. Start with guided meditation and let it take you from there. I have included videos on that aim to heal stress while focusing on the digestive system. You can find them at www.mysimplechanges.com/collections/stress-changes.

Meditation sounded so frivolous when a friend first told me about it. That's what "hippies" do, my preprogrammed thoughts would say. After again putting my ego to the side for the sake of healing, I leaped and committed to trying a ten-day free trial from a popular phone app. After just ten days of five minutes a day, I could feel the tightly wrapped, anxiety-filled areas opening and the stress triggers easing, not only healing my autoimmune disorder but healing my soul with its clarity, confirming its place and evolving one easier breath forward to lightening the autoimmune stronghold.

Meditation isn't new. In fact, it's thousands of years old. We're exposed to it more now that it's becoming more widely built into our fast-paced, consciously slowing down, efficiency-seeking lives. New to our ways, but there since the beginning in most cultures. Meditation works to regulate the amount of the hormone cortisol that's released into the system during times of stress. Cortisol evolves into inflammation-promoting chemicals called cytokines that initiate responses against inflammation and add fuel to the inflammation fire. Calming anxiety, reducing depression, and enhancing self-awareness through meditation blocks another path that collectively wears us within, by giving the overthinking, cluttered, distracted mind a chance to cool its head and offer a better approach to solutions.

Imagine walking along your favorite beach. The warm summer sun is shining and a cool breeze's gentle rolling rhythm is hitting your skin. As the waves crash and go, you feel the water at your feet. Each step forward leaves an imprint in the sand that slowly washes away as the distance grows. Now picture a rope around your torso tied to an anchor. It weighs more and more with each step forward you take. Then you see a shiny object in the sand ahead of you. It's a knife.

You pick it up and instinctively you know what to do. Cut the rope and leave the anchor behind to rust in the fading footsteps. As the tension releases, the sun's rays brighten. You continue on. Free. You take the deepest breath of a lifetime. Upon exhaling, you notice a figure walking toward you. It's a future version of you. You look healthy. Living the changes. Your future self smiles and thanks you for walking. You hug, squeezing tighter and lifting the weight from your shoulders, absorbing the changes before you let go and continue walking your beach. Step by step, you begin to realize why you were there, why you are here, and who you will become. All of that weight now gone.

Now imagine this story replaying in your mind while in your place of rest. The bed, the chair, the floor. That's our practice. That's our meditation. That's the release from the weight of the world's challenges. Calm yourself by giving yourself the freedom to see and cut the rope two or more times a day for at least ten minutes.

ESSENTIAL OILS

The mist in the room. A stress relief blend of an essential oil–filled diffuser. During meditation, yoga, dinner, or working, diffused essential oils can calm our toxic load. At this point in my progression, they replaced my deodorant, shampoo, body wash, lotions for sore muscles, rashes, itch relief, and to freshen up the carpets and floors. A good quality essential oil and blend like peppermint, eucalyptus, and tea tree not only avoids the harmful toxins we commonly use and absorb into our bodies through lotions and moisturizers, they also provide natural healing benefits.

The only precaution here is making sure to use a good, pure brand and blend for the particular condition. The science behind essential oils hasn't caught up to the trend and therefore makes us susceptible to oversaturated, low-quality product trials. Before going out and buying a variety pack and sticking them into every part of your life, invest in the purest, highest quality essential oil brands that avoid added carrier oils and harmful chemical processing that expose us to VOCs and other cancer-causing agents. The brands I've been using for a couple years now and recommend can be found on www.mysimplechanges.com/collections/all-products.

My Essential Oils Strategy (to start):

- Peppermint oil, lavender oil, tea tree oil, eucalyptus oil, clove oil, chamomile oil, rose oil, and frankincense for lotions and skin application.
- Peppermint, tea tree, rose, and clove for antifungal.
- Eucalyptus, frankincense, lavender, and chamomile for stress and anxiety.

Always pay careful attention to how your body reacts to each one. When science catches up, then let the decision expand, if warranted.

MASSAGES

Am I one of those people that asks for essential oils or brings in my own lotion to a massage? Yes, yes, I am. Health has no shyness, and that's the Simple Change. Why be shy about caring to the fullest extent of what *you* are exposed to?

Massages increase blood flow throughout the body, specifically in the brain, calming mood and regulating stress by aiding with the balance of cortisol levels and increasing the flow of feel-good chemicals like dopamine. Press deeper into the sympathetic nervous system, and massages decrease the creation of stress hormones in adrenal glands, which are a major factor in an imbalanced gut and autoimmune disease. The increase in blood flow establishes healthier cells by working to flush out the lymph nodes of any cells damaged by free radicals and an established toxic buildup. Also, they ease the pain, stress, and soreness we carry around unnecessarily.

A body of toxin-filled knots, formed from the postures and crippling of stress, can be broken up by the essential-oiled hands of a good massage therapist and flushed out through yoga, meditation, and water.

My Massage Tip: Work your way through different types of massages until you find the one suitable for your needs. Whatever works out the knots and allows the toxins to freely flush out, works for the changes. The pressure, style, and mood is up to you.

FOOD

At this point, we've figured out the foods we are allergic to, cleaned out obvious toxins from the home and common scenarios, made the stress changes, and yet we're still fighting to keep everything else in the diet that we can. I was determined to find any way possible to not have to give up meat, chocolate, and hangovers, even though I knew they were extremely tough for my body to process and filter. But progress is taking place and rounding out the last tactic for stress relief: food.

Certain foods help or hurt our stress and anxiety levels. That's widely understood. The ones that hurt are nowhere to be found in this book. Consider those to be the anxiety triggers. They're the ones that expose many other facets of our bodies.

Anxiety Triggers

- alcohol
- artificial flavors
- dairy
- lab-created ingredients
- natural flavors
- processed foods

My Anxiety-Calming Foods

- asparagus
- avocados
- berries
- chamomile flower tea
- dark chocolate (75 percent or darker and vegan)
- garlic
- leafy greens
- oranges
- oysters
- salmon
- turkey breast

Each of these foods works a different area of balancing and building to flush and restore your system from harmful chemical damage.

- Asparagus is rich in folic acid, which helps the body produce and maintain new cells and prevents damage to DNA (cancer loves damaged DNA).
- Avocados boost B vitamins (lost because of inability to absorb)—the same vitamins that build healthy nerves and brain cells—and help reverse a common deficiency associated with gut disorders (that leads to anxiety and tension in the system the more the deficiency worsens).

- Berries boost killer white blood cells by containing antioxidants and phytonutrients to reduce stress-related free radicals (commonly deficient with inflammation and autoimmunity).
- Chamomile flower tea regulates dopamine, serotonin, and apigenin, harmonizing excessive neurotransmitters and hormones in the mind while soothing the anxiously aware body.
- Garlic fights off oxidative stress in the same way as berries, with added punches of vital nutrients like manganese that also regulate stress.
- Leafy greens, well, we already know the multitude of essential mineral benefits of this main staple in the whole method success (easily digestible steamed or sautéed nutrient-rich greens).
- Oranges boost immunity with their vitamin C content, which lowers cortisol levels.
- Oysters and anxiety go shell in hand due to oysters' high protein and rich content of vitamins C and B12, iron, zinc, and selenium (plus libido, but we've all heard that one already).
- Salmon is loaded with omega-3 fatty acids that produce anti-inflammatory responses to regulate the negative effects of stress hormones (C-reactive protein tests reveal inflammation throughout the body, and omegas aid with the calming).
- Turkey breast and other meats help produce serotonin to regulate digestion, sleep, mood, depression, and memory (all affected from the leaking within, aka leaky gut).
- Dark chocolate unfortunately is one that needs to be skipped until fully healed (explained in the final chapter). Then, and

only then, reintroduce in small, periodic amounts for its micronutrient antioxidants, polyphenols.

It took a year after my grandmother's passing to build this framework. A year of working those five simple stress changes into my routine (yoga, meditation, essential oils, massages, and food) while continuing forward with understanding life and the toxic load I was still carrying. A year of commitment to understanding the stress that had plagued every day prior. Stress, that no matter how many food and supplement changes we make, still holds the ace of spades in the card game of autoimmunity.

This is a lot to remember. I understand. Grasp what connects. Memorize the yes foods, grow with the details. It gets easier with time and the reforming of routines into memory.

PART III: Exercise

CHANGING THE LOGIC: Finding Balance

There is a perpetual need to want the solution now. To get it all back at once. To be healed today, not tomorrow, but that mindset leads to overeating, overconsuming supplements, overstressing, and taking to heart the comments people are forever going to make. Forget what you look like on the outside, how skinny or fat or imperfect you think the world sees you. Those people are no longer your space. Focus on your gut and providing it the right balance. Every time I trip up is when I'm doing too much because of some perception I'm trying to achieve. The mindset is healing the body, and everything else falls into place from there. Stay focused on the principles of making the Simple Changes and trust that time will evolve them. Regardless of how the world speaks.

"You're so skinny. Are you feeling ok? Eat a carrot. Eat a steak. Did you lose weight? Do a pushup. When I hug you, I feel nothing. You're just bones." The quick skinny on the endless statements that turn into insecurities, of not being able to gain weight because the body doesn't absorb nutrients properly. The good thing is, the now is on healing and with healing comes healthy weight.

During the industrial revolution, the majority of us stopped simply surviving and started living for the most convenient lifestyle. As products have made our world more accessible, mindsets changed and survival of the fittest shifted to comfortable convenience. A continued goal today and every day. Until it affects our health. Then it's an issue. The avoidance of movement for ease of accessibility? Detrimental.

"More worthless than tits on a boar hog." One of Dad's favorites.

Don't be that worthless. Find the perfect balance of getting enough healthy movement, without overdoing it and causing more harm to digestion than good. The days of outrunning the suffering are a treadmill's revolving mat behind us. From the progression of waking up to a college hangover, to morning digestion stretches and biking through the beach day with her, to here, stretching and exercising as an unconscious conscious routine. My Simple Change's evolution of a healing habit.

With any exercise comes the need for ample stretching throughout the day. Morning digestion-focused stretches, before a workout stretches, or during a break from the work grind stretches. Be conscious of posture and take every chance during the day to "stretch it out" to bring increased blood circulation to rid the tissue of byproducts, increase flexibility to build stronger posture, and lessen tension throughout the body. Stretching also relieves the traffic jam of toxins piling up in our most vital parts, flushing them out and taking pressure off the gut. So, reach out, clear doubt, and breathe into that expansion.

Now that a good stretch has been had, and before movement begins, keep in mind that overindulgence, overexertion, or over anything leads to an imbalance that negatively affects the microbiome and branches out from there.

My Exercise Tips:

- To start off, never eat before exercising. Those are two different body functions and they should happen a couple of hours apart from one another. Trying to get all the good in at once can be just as bad as if not properly carried out.

- During exercise, be aware of overexertion. Overexertion causes damage to intestinal cell lining, which in turn breaks down the cells, reduces pressure in the colon, and releases harmful toxins into the bloodstream, causing food to move, or flush, out of the body quicker. Any stress or poor diet brought into the workout, mixed with rigorous activity and severely decreased blood flow, creates the same result, ridding the bowels of essential bile, microbes, and acid that now need to be rebuilt. Again. Back to square one. Different route, same wearing results. Same wearing results, increased risk for dehydration.

- Flush out or not, water intake needs to increase the more we get going. That's obvious, but dehydration is one of the main causes for exercise-induced gastrointestinal issues, and the more purified water you can give your body, the more soundly it will function.

- Variety. This is one of the biggest principles in exercise success. In fact, every aspect of the changes benefits from the widest range of variety. With exercise, it's that "thirty minutes a day is all you need, in a stress-calming place, to get it in and not overextend" kind of workout. Besides the firming of muscles for posture and abdominal support, or increasing blood flow for cleansing by adding a bit of "new blood" throughout, the right exertion daily increases heart rate. That is followed by a reduction in intestinal sluggishness, and an uptick in muscle stimulation—the good kind. Proper exercise also improves gut flora, essential to rebuilding the microbiome by repopulating its trillions of different microbes. Better gut flora smothers the growth of bad bacteria and aids with enzymes and acids to digest and absorb nutrients as they pass along the digestive tract.

Picture this with the other changes you have already built into the routine, mixed with the supplements and diet we'll cover in the last chapter, and you have a new team, a new space, and a new set of skills for your reformed foundation.

Before even taking that first step into "I'm going to finally commit" mode, identify throughout the day when you could take the stairs or walk to the store. Bike, hike, breathe, walk, sports, run, yoga, explore, and see your way into exercise. This space we've been constructing includes the quarter-mile walk to the grocery store. (A healthy relief after the years of sprinting through the sliding glass doors.) Or a bike ride through the countryside or along the shore. A hike for fresh air and clear mind while absorbing the views. Surround your space with routines that make exercise excitingly accessible. Get out of that small gym, running into the grey wall, with CNN on the TV and thoughts clouding the mind, and into the spaces where life speaks while exercise sneaks its way into healing.

PART II.I: Stress (cont.)

CHANGING THE LOGIC: *Resolve the Unresolved*

You read that heading right. We still have some unresolved to solve concerning stress. Techniques and exercise can only release so much. If you don't resolve the unresolved, you have nothing. That unresolved plagues the subconscious, and until peace is found it'll always creep its way back into autoimmunity, time and time again.

Confusion, anger, childhood shaping, trauma, relationships, family, misjudgments, and everything else that's swept under the rug, thinking they'll just go away, eventually forms mountains for us to trip over or stub our toe on. Finding that peace within by resolving the unresolved and moving forward is essential for that cortisol drip, and for our soul's peace. We can change all the food, add in every stress-relief strategy there is, and balance exercise, but if we're still surrounded by the unresolved, we'll never make it out.

"Why do you hold on to so much? Can't you just let that go?" Easy to say. But say those breaths into a mirror and watch them fog your self-reflection. We all have something to solve. Simple or extreme, it's there, and, as a result of it being there, the immune system suffers.

What controls us? That's a good place to start. How much of our stress controls who we are? How much of our life controls our stress? How much losing control does it take to let go?

Stress is something I still struggle with. It's still my biggest worst enemy (other than chocolate and that overeating thing). The only difference is, it doesn't win anymore. It doesn't destroy the paradise

I've built within and am constantly mindful of strengthening and reshaping. We're human. Not superhuman. No matter how much we like to think we are, we still feel and are going to feel and be confused about the "various" until the day we pass on. "He's my sensitive friend." I used to always resent that until recently becoming comfortable in realizing that I *do* feel more than others. Life has forced me to feel more than others. Through understanding came peace.

Our cells hear and listen to every thought and emotion. If the thoughts and trauma remain in the same space, our cells either build up or break down, taking extended time to regenerate while shortening our years of life. The effects of overstimulation releases cortisol (see the trend?) and chemicals throughout the body, throwing us into emotional cravings and spiraling from there. Everything we do or think or see or exist with is connected. Our body is so complex that, subconsciously or not, what we are consumed by ripples into every other area of our lives, internally and externally. These unresolved patterns take that cortisol and, like a broken faucet, continuously drip into our roots until we shut it off.

RESOLVE THE UNRESOLVED

In 2017, the expanding road of a healing commitment started to divide a partnership's once-energetic bond. Our happy home hit its point of detachment between the extent of changes I wanted to make and the ones that could not be parted ways with. It was all part of the multitude of things that takes its toll on a once-optimistic and adventurous companionship. People grow, people change, and people have great relationships in the detrimental but fun aspects of life, like food comas and nights that lead to missed-day hangovers.

Ultimately, my commitment to an entirely healthy space around a life I needed for healing took a toll on a relationship still holding on to the bar of "bottomless" habits. Loss creates pain that only time and a new space can heal. Healing can only happen by understanding how to let go. From this relationship I learned it's much more productive to finally let someone in and to love, than hide in the isolation of trying to figure it out alone. She showed me there was light through the darkness and that no matter who we were in the past, or what the world did to us, we have to find that peace or it will forever get in the way of what we want to keep. *Unresolved, resolved.*

Speaking of the bar. At this point, Dad was in the process of bringing new life to his. After over a decade, the same ol' was slowing down. Time for some spice. Through his adversities, and Grandpa Godsey now fading fast in his dementia, Dad stayed focused and balanced, rebuilding the restaurant into something fresh, giving it revitalized vibrancy. Every step along the way, I would hear people tell him what he should do to his restaurant. What would improve it. The food, the bands, the atmosphere—you name it, someone had the perfect solution. Even me. Where I'm proud of him, and what I admire him for, is that he listened and was gracious but ultimately stuck to his gut— his vision. He didn't let other people's opinions stress him out of his decisions, despite the weight that the rest of life was providing. He had a plan, and through trial, error, and time, saw it out.

Our lives are like his restaurant. Sticking to our plan, staying balanced, and understanding it takes time, while remaining humble to the world's ideas and graciously considering each one. Rebuilding with purpose and knowing the rest is out of our control. *Unresolved, resolved.*

Give up all you give to others who give nothing back. Free up those precious seconds and put it into those who values your time. We waste countless thoughts and hours of the day focused on finding ways to get a response and a connection back that's more than likely dropped our call well before. It leaves us lost in the stress of the "out of our control," and that results in the body doing one of three things: suffering now, exposing later, or wearing down too soon. None of those allow us to wear that flower-patterned shirt while sipping nourishment from an umbrella-covered coconut, in our peace chair by the bay. Remember, your time is the most valuable thing in your life, and your good health gives you more time. Release the ones who already let go versions ago. They're not a part of this new space. These new changes. This healthier version of you. ***Unresolved, resolved.***

People once thought the earth was flat and would murder anyone who said otherwise. Thankfully, nobody murders us publicly for eating a different way and caring about our bodies. But the execution can still be stealthily done by blocking the mind, surroundings, and progress with enabling justifications (found throughout this book). These people are stuck in the understandings of old habits. Let them drive through that tunnel. That's their vision. It isn't our struggle to hold on to anymore. We know there's always more to explore. ***Unresolved, resolved.***

One by one I let go, and one by one the separation anxiety grew. The fear of change. The fear of being alone. The fear of fear. One thing I learned is that there are some people who are never going to see you other than as a single version of yourself. But that's never going to be you anymore. Life is the evolution of you, and you are blossoming into

162

a healthier version. Some may never be able to see that. Keep close the ones who evolve as you evolve, and let go of the ones who remain stuck in an old version of you left lifetimes ago. *Unresolved, resolved.*

Two things happen from all of this letting go: the pain of saying goodbye and the healing of mending fences with the ones who were meant to stay. There are many people who let me go because of who I was and the strain I put into their peace. I'm positive about it and sad to see a few leave. There are many versions of myself I am happy to not be anymore. Just as there are many aspects that are still a work in progress. Aspects I now value because of making peace with the situation. The biggest difference? Understanding who you were, who you're never going to be again, and who you are right now. The current best version of you. Reach out one more time, let it out, and the rest is up to their peace. *Unresolved, resolved.*

Some experiences in our lives we can control. Some we cannot. Others we don't realize how out of control they've become until much, much later. Our youth shapes us in so many ways. Parents and guardians can try to shelter us from as much as they can, but the elements are going to show up regardless. It's what builds our character as people. The problem comes when the uncontrollable defines us.

It was fifth grade, midday, when my teacher softly leaned down and said to me, "Your mom wants you to go to the Adams family's house after school. They won't be home until late tonight." A little odd but not impossible. The Adams were neighbors, not Lurch and Morticia. My teacher being extremely friendly was unusual and nearly impossible. The day prior I had spent the afternoon working on math in the

163

principal's office and standing on the wall during recess. When I went to my friend's house after school, I remember thinking, "Why is his mom also being so nice?" Remember, I was a terrorizing "little shit" as my aunt still calls me.

A couple of hours later, my brother's girlfriend picked me up and we went home. She asked if I wanted to shoot hoops. Which was also strange. I spent thousands of hours shooting under the lights, but usually alone. We played as the setting sun changed to dusk's dark and car lights turned up the driveway, brightening with their approach. My dad got out of the Suburban. From his demeanor, I already knew. I froze as he walked closer, and through subconscious instinct said, "Did Grandpa die?" Now standing in front of me, he said, "Yeah, buddy." Shock turned and I instinctively started running from the pain. My heart pumped the body numb. Confusion kicked and broke the neighbors' compost bin. "How could he be gone?" That was my first understood experience with death.

For nearly two decades I struggled with his passing. It held a heavy, heavy weight inside me. He was a tough man. He had fought in the Battle of the Bulge during WWII and was forced to do unthinkable things during his time in the war. He earned a bronze star for his bravery when he and another soldier held the line while his platoon escaped with a group of POWs. The rest of his life was shaped by that time, channeled through his habits of alcohol and tobacco, hiding in his hurt and comedic personality. Despite it all, he was a great man and a loving grandfather. As a kid, I loved seeing Grandpa with his ever-present pipe in his mouth. As an adult, I realized that's *because* I always saw Grandpa with that pipe in his mouth. Ultimately, it gave him mouth cancer that spread to his lungs. But after all he had

164

survived, lung cancer wasn't going to be the thing that took him. So, he took himself shortly before. With the German Luger he gained from surviving the fight.

For eighteen years I struggled to understand why he would do that. Even in the darkest of times where I wanted the same solution for myself. I may not agree with what he did, which is why I struggled with it for so long, but I agree with the man he was to me and the pride he had for not wanting to suffer his way to the end. I finally understood the channeling he lived because of the battles he survived. From that came peace. Different set of circumstances and growth but connected in the parallel. I no longer want the same for myself. No more suffering until the end. ***Unresolved, resolved.***

Lastly, the more healing I've done and the better I've felt, the more I realize how much of my life was controlled by disease. I lived with it for so long it wasn't a part of me, but yet was me. Decades of never feeling sorry about the conditions because I just accepted them as my existence. I never thought about it or even used it as a justification, until I was free from its grips. I see why someone would feel sympathy now. I feel sympathy now. It's much easier to see someone else living a destructive path than our own, and it's much easier to say than to do. The less destructive it has become, the more pain I've felt from watching loved ones self-destruct their way to a shortened ending.

All of that time and energy spent at their side through the cancers and hospitals and yet-to-be-known results of Russian roulette, only for them to stubbornly ignore everyone around them and continue on the same path. Maybe some of this is survivor's guilt, or love's hurting heart. Nonetheless, no matter what healthy space we develop into, or the changes we make in the hope of encouraging their own improvement, it still carries the same weight. Because we are real, we love them, and we're built to feel emotions. It's easier to observe than reflect, and no matter how positive encouragement's intentions are, self-reflection is the only answer. This one is still a work in progress. **Resolve, still unresolved.**

CHAPTER 11: Mental Health

CHANGING THE LOGIC: Don't. Give. Up.

It's the biggest challenge of your life and will push your thoughts to the brink and cause you to question every single observance. Your unique circumstances that wear out hope. Wherever you are, whatever you're going through, keep searching. It is here, and it is out there, and as long as you're living, giving up is not an option.

This isn't necessarily a part I'd like to share. Not because I'm ashamed, but because of the instant judgment when telling someone. "He has depression. Stay away. Nobody has time for that," a girlfriend's father once said about someone. Unbeknownst to him, I have suffered a lifetime of depression and was going through it at that very moment. I felt so ashamed and she knew.

"Depression isn't something you can control, Dad." Loudly giving it back to him and quietly standing up for me. The perception is real and so is the illness. I wish I had never been affected by it or still feel the onset of it at times. Unfortunately, it's a sad truth the disease brings when the body is constantly deprived of nutrients and clarity.

Roughly 10 percent of our species suffers from massive depressive disorder (MDD) each year. Another vast majority fight through undiagnosed depression every day. The last majority have worn to it at least once over the course of a lifetime. In the three main areas of the brain, depression either shrinks or swells cell function, releasing or absorbing the dangerous chemical cortisol. Cortisol is released from the center of the brain, the hippocampus, and dispersed throughout the body. Cortisol within the hippocampus inhibits new neurons used for memory. When cortisol hits the front part of the brain, the prefrontal cortex, it shrinks the amount of memories, emotions, and decisions we can comprehend. Expanding through the last third of the brain, the amygdala, it disrupts sleep, routines, and emotional responses, ultimately evolving into sadness, depression, MDD, and suicide.

I'll admit. For decades I fought depression and suicidal thoughts.

Growing up, I was hyper, ate too much sugar, talked a lot, cried a lot, was annoying, a pain in the ass, cocky, insincere, too sensitive, and spoiled. I chased a lot of babysitters around with knives and locked them out of the house. Ok, that last sentence was true. The rest was said by various people for various reasons that are out of my control. Constantly, I listened to those people and let it build. Maybe I was that way. Maybe I wasn't. What I was though, was a defenseless body exposed to being severely affected by anything. My vulnerability was easy to prey on. All those opinions continuously piled onto one another, starting with me being my own worst critic and eventually evolving into no longer wanting to live.

Mental illness isn't an illness. It's an effect of a rooted cause. Roots that also grow Crohn's disease. Autoimmune disorders. Deficiencies. Mental stress from not feeling well, or from feeling too much, rooted outward from the diseased brain of an already weakened immune system and microbiome. A digestive system unable to properly absorb nutrients cuts off supply to sufficiently feed the brain and, in turn, signals the rest of the body to panic and dry up any logical clarity. Sensitizing words worsen the condition. The depletion expands. Stress from the Crohn's disease, stress from the side effects of steroids and other medicines, stress from being constantly tired, stress from missing life, stress from nobody understanding, stress from being trapped in a place I knew I didn't want to spend another minute in but had no idea how to get out of, stress from years of misrepresentation because the presentation was not the truth of who I was, and stress unresolved.

As my health deteriorated throughout my youth and the negative thoughts grew louder, the rabbit hole kept burrowing into depression. College, that freedom-fest and great time in life, proved to be the worst time to not be mentally strong. New environment, new friends, new routines, new insecurities, new habits, and added stress to the mental melting. The confusion and feelings of youth took advantage, and a teenager's understanding of suicide paralleled the growing justification of it being a reasonable decision. We all have to walk the sad truths of life. The way we digest it is what creates our peace. At that point in my life, I was done digesting.

The simplest of tasks become the hardest of movements. Constant flushing of the body left my energy exhausted. Medicine and diseased digestion invited the most nauseated of times. The world looked angry. The person in the mirror was ugly. "Nobody would miss you. Those things they've said? It's all true." That's not who I am. Why can't I get rid of this person? Why won't anyone hear me? Listen to me? Where'd everyone go? When I need them the most. Nobody cares. Nobody's there. I don't feel well. I hate this. What is there left to do? I've tried everything. I don't want to be here anymore. I can't do this anymore. Why live? Goodbye.

Suicide is not the fact of wanting to kill yourself; it's the only seemingly logical escape when you can no longer live in the torment. I tried to escape a couple of times. Threatened it a few more. Thought about it constantly. Talked to professionals, took the calming drugs, hid in the shadows, and remained frozen in the idea of what the normal says is "normal" and to "deal with it." I stood on the ledge until Grandma Godsey passed quietly in her sleep. Her lasting impression forced me to take a step back, and the escape about-faced and walked toward the solution. With disease, imbalance, and diminution comes depression.

My Depression Tips: Take any such thoughts and force the about-face. Put your weight of trust into yoga, meditation, exploring, and exercising to calm, to allow the toxins to leave, and the allergies and food changes to heal. You're not alone. At least one person understands. Me.

Also, lean on the changes, lean on the support system, lean on something. Standing tall on the outside while living broken within keeps the situation broken. As progress happens with the food changes and relieving the pressure of your toxic load, clarity finds its way through the darkness. Step into the habits of your needed stress-relief changes. As you make headway, the tension slowly releases and the deception of the day paints color. The mind heals as the gut heals. The autoimmunity or ailments heal as the gut heals. Calming, patching, rebuilding, and sustaining. Surround every part of the day with the positive thoughts and actions needed to step a little easier. No matter how hard it is, step and don't give up. Never give up. Movement eventually reveals light and you will find your laughter again.

Do I still get depressed today? Of course. We all go through it. Do I get to those levels anymore? Not even close, and if the thought even comes into my mind, I can now identify what is missing from the balance and meditate for the answer. This sounds so easy. Right? And it is, because you are not alone anymore. Whenever you hit that point in your life where the sadness is winning, find the restore somewhere in this method. I don't want you to go. The world doesn't want you to go. You don't want you to go. You just haven't found the way back to your purpose yet. Food, stress relief, exercise. Heal to feed the brain and in return the brain will feed the body with the right messages. Walk, hike, disconnect, go, see, talk, get it out. A step is all that is needed to start. Scratch, claw, bite, will your way through that step. Whatever it takes. Once stepping starts, so does evolving. And always remember, it's not your fault for feeling the way you do. But it is, if you go.

CHAPTER 12: Today

NILES, MI - Austin Godsey, Jr., 89, passed away at 8:15 pm on Monday, January 1, 2018 at Rittenhouse in Michigan City, IN.

Austin was born on January 10, 1928 in Martinsville, IN to the late Minor and Flossie (McDaniel) Godsey, Sr. On April 8, 1952, Austin married Marilyn (McCoy) and she passed away on May 10, 2016, after 64 years of marriage...

It was actually 3:30 p.m. When he fought with the last he had, to stay until his son arrived bedside. At that point, he was down to a whisper. "Where's Mark?" My dad was thirty minutes away, rushing from Joey Armadillo's to get there, as my mom and I held him. Dementia may have taken most of his final days, but he was present in his last moments. By the time my dad arrived, Grandpa had stopped speaking. Love through his calm blue eyes was their final connection. His son brought him peace, and we held each other as we watched his brain shut down. At 8:15 p.m., the rest of him turned off as well. My best friend was my grandpa. My dad's best friend was his dad. The best man I've ever known was the only person I've heard spoken about the same way, by everyone.

Six months earlier, she went one way and I went another, our days on the bay ended. A once love-filled relationship now forever left in a time, leaving me homeless and fixated on making my new endeavor work. I got lost and lost myself in the exertion, which developed into an obsession to prove myself right and to fulfill a purpose of helping others. There were many problems with the routes I was taking to heal the pain of them and finishing what I started with this undertaking, and all were now exposed.

Shortly before our split, my dad fought through bladder cancer, and around the same time, we lost Grandma Godsey.

On January 1st, 2018, at 8:15 p.m., when that final call came to my father, the pain, the losses, and the experience of seeing Grandpa go forced thousands of hours of hard work past its breaking point and into a desperate decline. While I walked Michigan's brisk winter shoreline looking for clarity, I thought, "Nothing else matters anymore." Through the bitter cold to the library, "Anything without life isn't real." From sunshine to freezing rain and home to the coffee shop, "Everything else is made up." Detaching to reattach, "The people and the walk are all that matters." These days in isolation are where I found value.

Living an imbalanced life of sleeping in a car while overworking beyond exhaustion, you get collapse. That triggered desperation, over-supplementation and a panicked plea for immediate relief. Fuel added to a smoldering fire. I lost sight of the methods that healed me in the first place. There was too much to comprehend at once to logically understand how my body was feeling. Through the months of walking and sorting, the next questions rang. "What am I going to do? Maybe everyone was right? Maybe I can't heal this disease? Should I just give up? Give in?"

The thing about taking steps forward is, eventually you've taken so many your only choice is to get up and start stepping again, from the place you've fallen to. From today. Gone astray I was because of life's inevitable. Enough changes I had built into my routine to know I had the strength to finish the healing and finally prove I could put the disease into remission.

"Ok, so how am I going to do this?" By going back to the basics of My Simple Changes and making the proper appointments, figuring out exactly what was going on, growing through this evolved condition's understanding, and working the core routines. Taking control once more, knowing it's going to take time, but that success will be had. Building and fighting and overcoming. Again.

Leaving only the final piece to the peace. Or peace to the piece. Both.

CHANGING THE LOGIC: Enjoying Good Days, Accepting Bad Days

There are going to be good days. There are going to be bad days. There's going to be progress. There's going to be relapse. The best we can do is be consciously aware at all times and calm to an understanding of what's lacking. Acknowledge the progress that's been made and fully immerse into the relief strategies built from previous chapters. Temptations are always going to try and justify their way into short-term decisions the more vulnerability grows. The deeper invested in the changes we are, the easier it is to give ourselves the space and time needed to balance before breakdown.

In my twenties, I always wanted to be everything. Through wanting to be everything, I never held on to anything. Now, in my thirties, I just want to be something. By wanting to be something I let go of everything. Youth gave me experience and retrospect's understanding, college broke the limits, shingles broke the deadly cycle, the day on the bay built a new diet and toxin-relief foundation, Grandma Godsey's death rebuilt my brain by learning movement and breath, and Grandpa Godsey reset everything to finally find my something.

My 'Back to the Beginning' Tips (recapping & expanding):

- First, set up the proper appointments with doctors who care about you, the individual. Start with a primary care physician and work outward. A dermatologist, gastroenterologist, internal medicine doctor, or any other specialist needed for the suspected conditions.

- Next, don't for a second ever feel ashamed for caring about the full extent of your health. This is a daunting task. I get it. I hate anything medical when it pertains to me and the thought of going through even the simplest parts of the process. But this is where you dig deep and will yourself into getting the answers you need. For every detail. All the way to finding the yoga class where a good yogi brings relaxation to the practice. To a massage therapist who understands your condition and goals. Or a therapist who can help resolve the unresolved. It doesn't have to be a professional therapist, or even a person for that matter, just an outlet for putting peace to the trauma. Like my first choice, meditation. Always, and often. It's the easiest to do and probably the most beneficial for all states of healing. Next thing I choose, being outside. Away from the noise. Somewhere new. For calm and clarity.

- When you finally make it into the room with the doctors, be honest about your condition, symptoms, and goals. If they show any tunnel vision routines or still oppose you after you've explained your desire for tests to figure out inflammation levels, infections, and deficiencies, then you need to find another doctor. Approach this while showing respect. They're people too, and so are their staff. More respect, more response. More response, more answers. More answers, more solutions. More solutions, more time alive. Also, know what your insurance covers and how you can get the most from your doctors to get the needed work done. A full body scan is ideal, to assure how every system is running and processing. Fecal matter tests, blood food allergy tests, deficiencies, fungus, infections, inflammation, viruses, bacteria, yeasts, heavy metals, polyps, cancer, and everything safely possible within modern technology. Especially the ones associated with autoimmunity and your suffering microbiome. If you're not already following the changes outlined, the diet laid out, and living in an eco-friendly bunker far underground, you are affected by modern times and owe it to yourself to assess the full extent of how your body is holding up. Waiting until later only subjects you to worsened conditions.

- Then, keep a file of every result, your entire medical history. This is your health journey, and the more information you and the team have, the easier it is to understand what's within the markers and what's not. The power to see progress, or regression, is in your hands.

If finances are still the issue, and understandably so, continue to follow the changes and diet, because they will help. At the very least, they'll help you gain a better understanding for yourself and what's going on. But don't let finances be a justification. The first time I was admitted to the ER during "the house collapses," I didn't have insurance or a plan. I was sick, I needed help, and I went to the emergency room. The second time, fear of the bills that were coming, fear of not knowing how I was going to pay, left me in a spiraling decline until losing control of my thoughts in those "blood- and sweat-soaked clothes." When I still held clarity, the bills were scary. But in the end, they were going to be whatever they were. Money is a made-up thing. The price of your life is more valuable than anything. Go, fight, and figure out a way to get the care you need. With the technology we have today and the ease in our overall quality of life, there's no reason to let our pains linger anymore.

When I was seventeen, I suffered a severe pinpricking pain in my abdomen during a drill at soccer practice that sent my dad and me to the ER. The doctor at the time believed I was suffering from an overgrowth of yeast in my intestines. It was never made official and I didn't think twice about yeast or hear about it as an issue for the next fifteen years. Overactive yeast, infection, fungus, parasites, or similar ended up being one of the underlying causes of my conditions. Fifteen years it took for me to find the connections between the deficiency and overgrowth in the intestines. A hidden factor that lingered, sickened me, and worsened over time.

In 2018, the understanding of overgrowths in our gastrointestinal tract and how they are key factors in our structural declines are coming to light. The conditions we are exposed to through lifestyle and diet create habitable situations for these overgrowths, and most of our standard tests don't even hint at registering these possibilities; the ones that do are limited in their understanding of the significance. This is another reason to run all tests associated with the immune system and gut while having a team that understands the widest range of scientific possibility. In time, more will become known about it, but for now, and for always, be proactive while still keeping as much of an outsider's observance as logically possible.

05/09/2018

VISIT TYPE:

Preventive Medicine

This 33-year-old male presents for preventive exam and Crohn's.

History of Present Illness:

1. Crohn's

The symptoms began 11 years ago. The symptoms are reported as being moderate. The symptoms occur randomly. He states the symptoms are chronic and are in remission. Diagnosed in 2007. Had colectomy in 2010. Was treated with Remicade 4 years ago. No recent flare ups.

MARITAL STATUS/FAMILY/SOCIAL SUPPORT

Currently single. Does not have children.

Patient's support network includes father, friends and mother.

SMOKING STATUS

Never smoker

ALCOHOL

There is a history of alcohol use.

(Now) consumed rarely.

CAFFEINE

The patient does not use caffeine.

VITAMIN D TOTAL

16 ng/mL L

Deficiency

<20 ng/mL

Patient Plan

I will request authorization for Gastroenterologist.

The month-long wait for my PCP appointment led to another month for a GI appointment and finished the process of procedures three weeks later (nearly three months total). When I sat in a pre-operation room lined with occupied beds and divided by curtains awaiting my colonoscopy and endoscopy, I heard a first-timer telling the nurse he was nervous about his colonoscopy. She went on to say, "You're doing the right thing by being proactive and getting checked before it's too late." Which is 100 percent correct. Given the state of our digestive epidemic, waiting until fifty is too old. She then went on to say, "Everyone will tell you to eat organic, but this is genetics. Organic and diet doesn't change genetics."

There's the disconnect.

We need every form of medicine, and it's nobody's fault but the person who doesn't hear all opinions before forming solutions. I felt my disease was in remission. But everyone, even the PCP and my closest family, doubted it. "He (the patient) states the symptoms are chronic and in remission." Or, "Does he really think he can cure it?" I heard this constantly and because of it, at times I doubted myself as well. Despite all the signs and improvements of my symptoms, regularly being surrounded by a rising brow will make you feel crazy and overthink every slight pain, irregularity, or mishap. Ultimately, that keeps you in the sickness. When all that's ever been spoken is, "there isn't a cure," nobody will believe progress until it's proven, which makes it easy for justifications to revive and doubt to take over. But you know what? Forget them. This is you. Us. And it works.

"Mr. Godsey, it's time for your colonoscopy. Are you ready?"

I was patient six of nearly thirty that morning receiving colonoscopies by the same doctor. This ought to be good.

"More than you'll ever know, ma'am."

Quietly, I was scared of the results. What if they were right and the Crohn's was still there? What if it was worse? What if? What if? What if?

During my post-op revitalization, I was offered apple juice and graham cracker cookies. I'm allergic to apples and gluten and would rather not step further back with the other substances in that toxic pack of cookies. I asked for a different juice. Cranberry came and so did sugar, corn syrup, soy lecithin, artificial flavors, and the gang of words the general population has no clue how to pronounce but irritate the lining of our guts and weaken our immune system. The front of the label did tell me it was a good source of calcium though. Like that cute bunny on the carton of chocolate milk, hospital food is ordered from the same salesmen that fill those Styrofoam lunch trays and load those restaurant freezers, furthering the disconnect between Western medicine, holistic medicine, and Eastern medicine.

Despite that, all the tests were run, appointments came and went, and now it was the waiting game. When those scary results do finally come, it's not the end of the world. Even if they show the end of our timeline, they still provide answers and options. We tend to not explore the possibilities because keeping a distance justifies an irrational peace, which leads to the acceptance of ignoring our duty to ourselves. Whatever the probability is, identify it, face it, embrace it, and treat it.

Understanding the Results Tips: Start by keeping a space that promotes rational decisions for the course of action. Then, lean on the support system, discuss with the A-team, and fall back on the My Simple Changes foundation, while keeping in mind all we now know about the gut and the main goal of building without compromise. Functional medicine uses the body's natural processes to heal. Western medicine uses drugs. Eastern, herbs. Education finds routes for our specific healing. Explore the education of your conditions using all methods of medicine available. Knowledge is a healthy person's power.

Even before all of your issues have been identified, despite the results, I can already tell you that it's time to go on a strict anti-inflammatory diet of my simple recommended foods that avoid triggers, allow the bowel to rest, and reset the microbiome bacterium.

MY SIMPLE LIST OF INFLAMMATION-HEALING FOODS
Purified water **(very important)**
FRUITS

Blueberries	Pineapple
Cherries	Raspberries
Coconut yogurt	Strawberries
Oranges	Tangerines

VEGETABLES

Any leafy green	Bok choy
Artichokes	Broccoli
Arugula	Brussels sprouts
Asian mushrooms	Cabbage
Avocados	Carrots
Beets	Cauliflower

Celery	Leeks
Chard	Maca
Collard greens	Onions
Garlic	Spinach
Kale	Sweet potatoes (all variety)

MEATS (most important)

Bone broth	Salmon
Lean, grass-fed meats	Sardines
Oysters	

SPICES

Basil	Raw honey (only topical)
Cinnamon	Rosemary
Cloves	Sage
Ginger (fresh or powder)	Thyme
Olives (cans: water & salt)	Turmeric (fresh & powder)
Oregano	

OILS

Coconut oil

Olive oil

MY SIMPLE LIST OF INFLAMMATION TRIGGERS

Alcohol	Low-quality or excessive
Chicken (anything but the very	amounts of red meat
best)	Margarine
Dairy	Vegetable oils (corn,
Fried foods	safflower/sunflower, soybean,
Fruit juices	peanut, cottonseed)
High-glycemic index foods	Processed foods
(sugar and grains)	Salt

Soda or sugar-sweetened
drinks (any)

My Simple Lists are mere suggestions and a foundational guideline. Your specific conditions may be different. Remember that, and give yourself the time, sleep, peace, water, movement, and attention you need and deserve. Avoid personal triggers and common inflammatory ones, like nightshades, alcohol, high glycemic fruits, and grains.

When deciding on each substance to consume remember, ten good qualities is easily negated by one bad. Just because a random website says that aloe juice and slippery elm are good for inflammation, or fermented foods are good for probiotics, it doesn't mean it's time to jump into an every-serving overindulgence. Too much of anything is not a good thing, and while healthy gut substances like slippery elm and aloe may have calming effects by supporting the building of healthy mucus in the gut, they also have immune response capabilities and commonly trigger symptoms. Debated or negatively proven substances fall under the same restrictions. Sticking to the positively established is the solution. With fermented foods, a healthy rotation is the balance; every meal is an overindulgence. Minimal, if at all while healing bacteria overgrowth, is my recommendation. Wait until balance has been restored before slowly incorporating fermented foods back into your diet. Avoid this common mistake by taking into consideration everything each ingredient provides and consuming only the entirely good substances varying in proportion to your current condition.

Because the most important thing is life. The most important thing to life is health. The most important thing for health is commitment.

These changes are sometimes not going to feel good. In the first couple of weeks you'll feel bloated, stocked up, and like something is wrong. It's going to be uncomfortable. But you know what else is uncomfortable? This entire story. My story. Your story. The sickness in our story. The unruly misfits are not being fed; they're dying off and the rest of the microbiome is resetting from healthy cell regeneration. Commit the time and, in time, balance will come.

CHANGING THE LOGIC: Stress Starts at Home

Important to the progress of anything is a stable home life. Before her, my life was reckless and dark. A good woman brought balance. A good home brought routine. Routine brought more focus by lessening detrimental distractions. Fight for the peace of a stable living situation and environment. Your current situation may be bad, the worst, or below your standards, but it'll never change if you don't fight with the commitment of growing through the pain. A healthy space starts at home and healing the gut builds outward.

Going through my house today, the products, space, and food, you'll find it's filled with specifically chosen items that will keep me healthy enough to avoid having to spend another night in the hospital, or even the car for that matter. Following are My Simple Lists of those household changes. Keep in mind, our knowledge is always expanding. For the most up-to-date list of products I recommend, and use, please feel free to refer to https://mysimplechanges.com/collections/all-products.

In the home, you have to be conscious of the off-gassing or clever chemical killers in the carpet, rugs, paint, furniture, electronics,

185

fixtures, clothing, and every little thing that rapidly add up and derail progress. Being an artist, where being frugal is key, I have gone the route of buying years-old secondhand furniture that has had time to breathe off its manufacturing fumes. Otherwise, purchase products from a company that puts value into making us an eco-friendly, nontoxic product.

Common Household Toxin Scenarios: Our cotton, our wood, our fake wood, and every piece of purchased, doused, soaked, sprayed, and constructed with fire-retardant substances, bleaches, dyes, and other toxic fumes. Remember, we breathe all of those in and we spend on average more than half of our life at home.

The Bedroom

- Bed: Mattress, mattress pad, mattress protector, pillow stuffing and encasing, sheets, pillow cases, blankets and comforter, find all GOTS-certified organic cotton, bamboo, or wool. At the minimum, and in order, choose pillow, sheets, mattress pad. The maximum: all. Whatever you can afford, do. Doesn't have to be all at once. One thing at a time, over the course of time.
- Furniture: Night stands, lamps, chairs, rugs, dressers, shelves, bed frame, and whatever you put on the walls.
- Electronics: TV, computers, phones, clock, assistant devices, and everything else transmitting signals. Phone on airplane mode and everything else off unless using.
- Miscellaneous: Paint, carpet, floors, plants, airflow, Hepa air purifier, diffuser, lighting, and no scented candles.

Don't forget, upon waking up do digestion stretches and brush the teeth of any overnight bacteria buildup. Digestion starts in the mouth, and morning breath is a sign to remove those nasty toxins before they join the rest of the digestive tract and wear into greater infections.

"So, bring your bests, boys! Brandon, have a mint." Thanks then, no need now. There's nothing positive with mints or gum or candy beyond the immediate refreshing relief. Ridding yourself of those sugar-loaded, sugar-free, or fructose-plagued treats cuts off another supply to the invaders and homesteaders. Two root canals, four crowns, and one cavity later, I finally took initiative and fixed what grew from a dull ache to intense pain and a tooth infection that connected its way with my gut.

The Bathroom

- We already changed to a homemade essential oil deodorant, nontoxic hand soap, fluoride-free toothpaste, bamboo toothbrush, essential oil shampoo/soap, GOTS-certified organic cotton towel and wash cloths.
- Changes like, applying a whipped homemade blend of organic shea, unrefined coconut oil, and pure essential oil blend moisturizer to a freshly washed face. Or rinsing with a tablespoon of coconut oil and a drop of oregano oil, or clove oil to kill any invading bacteria.
- Switching to a nontoxic rug, purified shower water, nontoxic (including bleaches and dyes) toilet and tissue paper, and tea tree dental floss.

After that, heat up a cup of purified water for the first, much needed, liquids of the day. Leave the caffeine fix of coffee as yesterday's consumption. The antinutrients and caffeine in the bean can irritate gut lining and cause intestinal contractions that ultimately disrupts digestion. (Antinutrients are explained later in this chapter.) The majority of mornings I consume hot water, sometimes with lemon juice or collagen peptides; sometimes with ginger, lavender, and mint; and on the rarest of times any other approved tea, like peppermint. All rotated for their rich nutrients and their abilities to soothe the intestinal tract while lubricating the natural flow outward. There's no need to start the day off irritating the lining of the stomach, altering blood sugar levels, and forcing an imbalance of acidities. Especially before the first meal is even healthily consumed.

My First Meditation of the Day: While the world is still quiet, take advantage of the opportunity and give yourself the first meditation of the day. Ten to thirty minutes. For the clarity and strength we need for a day of logical decisions and reactions. Also, meditating before breakfast starts the drip of endorphins and quiets the crowd of cortisol and adrenaline. Happy mind, happy gut, and vice versa.

In this die off and resting time, the keys are liquids, relaxing the bowels, incorporating easily digestible nutrition, and balancing with supplements specific to tackling those allergies, infections, and raw dealings the body has been suffering through. So, twenty minutes before breakfast I usually take a digestive enzyme, to give my stomach extra assistance for the upcoming work. A full spectrum digestive enzyme pill that replaces what's been depleted.

Breakfast is all about efficiency and little effort. In order to make that happen, the kitchen needs to be efficiently stocked. Here's my list of those items and a recipe for the breakfast I most often consume:

The Kitchen

- Water filter for sink and ice. Dishwasher too, if possible. No fluoride or unwarranted added chemicals.

- Nontoxic pots and pans, utensils, storage containers, cups. Use stainless steel and glass as much as possible.

- Eliminate plastic anything. Minimize it from the products you buy and never reuse it. Always recycle. The plastic pollution problem is sadly real. Just take a walk on any one of our shorelines.

- BPA-free cans, pantry items of whole ingredients without any added substances that don't fall into the rest of the changes, and fresh herbs if possible.

MEAL #1: Sweet Potato Bowl

Ingredients

1 medium organic sweet potato (purple, orange, white, doesn't matter. Vary and rotate.)

½ cup (no more) fruit: banana, cranberries, or raspberries

1 tablespoon minced fresh organic ginger

1 tablespoon pineapple juice or maple syrup (optional, and only after symptoms have subsided)

1 tablespoon unrefined cold-pressed organic coconut oil (or coconut butter, milk, cream and flakes, without guar gum to avoid any possibilities of irritating the stomach's lining)

1 teaspoon ground cinnamon

1 teaspoon ground turmeric

¼ cup broccoli or kale microgreens, or sprouts (depending on balance of the day's remaining menu)

Instructions

Set the oven to 400°F.

Scrub the sweet potato. Dry it, place on a baking sheet, and bake until you can easily stick a fork through it, about 40 minutes.

While the sweet potato is baking, pour 1/3 cup of purified water into a pan on the stovetop. Bring to a simmer.

Add the cranberries, ginger, and the pineapple juice or maple syrup.

Simmer until the cranberries have absorbed the liquids.

In a bowl, butterfly and mash the sweet potato.

Top with the coconut oil, cinnamon, turmeric, and microgreens (or sprouts), and enjoy!

The average time we spend a day on our phones is two hours. Two hours a day for a year is a month of our life lost in a device. I like being on my phone, but at the end of the day, it's not healthy for people with a suffering immune system, and real life is being missed. My solution was to set up my most controlled space, the home, with distractions that keep me productive and don't waste any more valuable time.

Remaining Household Items to Consider:

- Hepa air purifier, air-cleansing plants, nontoxic rugs, carpet and paint, minimal electronics and off-gassing furniture, mass-produced anything, pillows and blankets.
- Cleaners: for vacuuming, sprinkle baking soda onto a carpet, spray with a diluted lavender oil essential oil blend, and let sit for an hour or so before normal vacuuming. This will help disinfect, refresh, and sweep away any collection, preventing it

from building into immune system–weakening issues like mold and the toxins that are constantly tracked and walked around the home. Only use cleaners that offer natural sources and are nontoxic to our health. (That includes bleach.)

CHANGING THE LOGIC: *Food Journal*

List the ingredients of every meal and grocery store needs in your phone, labeled My Dinner or My Breakfast or My Smoothie or My Groceries or My Whatever Gets You to Do It. It's easier to stay disciplined and stick to an appropriate meal when the list is actively planned into the day. There's no forgetting it at that point and it keeps your food freshly balanced, limits waste, and you'll be more efficient about spending because, again, preparing your food saves money. It also limits impulse junk food purchases and last-minute justification decisions. More importantly, you've now created a food journal to help better understand what foods have been consumed at different times, and what foods you may be consuming too much of for your current condition. Also, if illnesses develop, the list can aid in the solution. A simple task of just writing down a shopping list labeled for a quick search gives you a better grasp on your consumption patterns.

The progression of science in a Western society and the availability of endless forms of manufactured substances changed the way we eat. We haven't had the time to prepare for our health anymore. This morning's extra time for a day of eating is accomplished by yesterday's conscious planning and the prior day's commitment to making the changes, ultimately snapping lunch into glass containers and protecting us from another vulnerable moment of the outside world's landmines. Also, remember to pack that stainless steel (no plastic or polyurethane cap) bottle filled with filtered purified, or alkaline, water. I alternate between the two to help balance the body's acidities, or pH levels. Proper pH balance allows the body to produce adequate amounts of the bile, acids, and enzymes needed to break down foods and nutrients throughout the entire digestive tract. You can easily track your current levels, and progress, by spending just a few dollars and purchasing pH test strips.

Always remain conscious of consuming 50 to 64 ounces of water a day. One of my strategies is to fill two-gallon glass bottles (or approved thermos) at the grocery store or home filter and putting one in my car and one in a spot that I will see while home. In sight, in mind: positive change accomplished. For the rest, I take my stainless-steel bottle with me. Both make it easier to gauge daily consumption, avoid plastic leaching and unproperly treated water toxins from entering our bodies, save money (and the plastic-filled environment), and avoid commonly concocted "progress killer" drinks, like pop (or soda).

Now, the other work. Work, work.

"Wait, you didn't shower?"

This is true. Showering once or twice a day is what our bacteria-afraid culture trains us to do. "You might have gotten someone else's germs. Take a shower!" I learned early on that impure water and heat deplete the microbiome. One of my main focuses is keeping my body in an optimal state for good bacteria to survive and grow. We need every good soldier possible for this war. So, if the day didn't require it, then I probably didn't take it. Instead, I washed with a purified water–soaked cloth and soap or essential oil blend. Same short-term cleaning, healthier long-term result, and more money in my wallet. Because in the long run, it's cheaper. I also brushed my teeth for the second time of the morning. It's the last thing I do before lacing up my shoes and facing the day.

When I worked for the beverage company, days in the office went a little like this: "Another morning in paradise, Accounting Tom." Repeated for the 312th time. "Two days till Friday, Cindy!" Fake smiles all around. "Nine more hours." Landing at my thumbtacked photo- and document-lined corkboard cubicle. Sit. Exhale. Life. Wasted.

If anything about that paragraph sounds familiar, it's time to find your one shot at life a new profession. Work should be like coming home. Work should inspire us, not contribute to our cortisol drip. A third of life is our work. Is it a third of our stress? Or happiness? Our choice.

Regardless, whether you love or hate your work, you still have to take breaks. After two to three hours of focus, walking away, enjoying lunch, stretching and breathing in another space for even just a minute, releases the tension built from a half day of concentration, avoids the toxic roadblock caused by compression, and opens up the lung space before stress and anxiety tighten it off.

Roughly three hours after the first meal and before the second meal of the day, I try and get my second helping of stretching and at least ten minutes of meditation in.

Then I aim for a combination of these elements: leafy greens, colored vegetables, 4 to 6 ounces of meat protein, a healthy fat, spices, and some kind of fiber. Orange, purple, green, white, and yellow vegetables, rotated and painted in array with each meal. Remember: always sautéed or steamed, not the same leafy green as the last meal, but greens with every meal. Avoid overconsumption.

MEAL #2: Lettuce Cup Jackfruit (or Fish) Tacos

If you're in a rush, need variety, or want a simpler lunch, choose canned pink salmon or sardines, from a brand that tests for heavy metal content.

Ingredients

½ beet (roasted and thinly sliced)

1 can jackfruit (water and salt, no brine) or 1 can fish

¼ cup chopped leek

¼ cup Asian mushrooms (your choice)

¼ cup chopped celery

¼ cup chopped green olives

1 teaspoon unrefined/unfiltered extra-virgin olive oil

½ cup bone broth

1 tablespoon coconut aminos

1 teaspoon ground turmeric

1 (1-inch) piece fresh ginger, minced

1 tablespoon chopped fresh rosemary

1 teaspoon ground sage (or 1 tablespoon fresh, minced)

¼ avocado (sliced)

1 scallion (white and green parts, chopped)

3 to 5 butterhead lettuce cups

Instructions

Set the oven to 400°F.

Wash, dry, cut off the tips, cover in aluminum foil, and place the beets in the oven for 45 minutes or until soft, testing by poking with a fork. (Tip: I cook 3 or 4 beets and store the rest to make my meal planning easier.)

While the beets are cooking, strain the jackfruit and combine with the leek, mushrooms, celery, green olives, olive oil, bone broth, coconut aminos, turmeric, ginger, rosemary, and sage in an appropriate pan on the stovetop.

Turn the heat to medium and simmer while gently mixing and breaking up the jackfruit with a fork.

Simmer until the liquids have cooked off, 6 to 10 minutes, then place half in a glass container for lunch and the other half in a separate glass container for later.

When the beets have cooked, remove from the oven, peel, and slice.

Combine the avocado, sliced beet, and scallion and place on top of your lunch portion of jackfruit mixture.

Wrap your desired number of lettuce cups in a paper towel and place in a glass container.

Pack the appropriate condiments and smile for how simple that was!

Note: If using fish, simply omit the bone broth and jackfruit, and cook the same way.

"Why are we giving up all grains and seeds, again? They're healthy in even the most similar diets to yours!"

This is true. Nuts, seeds, grains, and legumes are healthy, when treated properly. Here it is. Just as animals have venom and poisons as a defense mechanism to deter predators from eating them, so do seeds, nuts, grains, legumes, and many other common foods.

195

Antinutrients like phytates, tannins, trypsin inhibitors, lectins (hemagglutinins), gluten, alkylresorcinols, oxalates, enzyme inhibitors, protease inhibitors, and alpha-amylase inhibitors make up the substance of defense against insects, predators (like humans), molds, and fungus. Once consumed into our digestive system, healthy body or not, they defend themselves the same way.

Picture opening anything that is sealed in hard plastic. It's sealed for a reason. In the same way, we need to remove these antinutrients to get to the present we intended with their purchase. They need to be treated and eradicated, by anything but our teeth, before being consumed. Any other way is a pipeline to agitation, deficiencies, and the rabbit hole of inflammation that wears us into autoimmunity. For the beginning repairing phase, these foods are completely eliminated from the diet because the risk is not worth the setback. They can only be reincorporated after the My Simple Changes and A-team plan has calmed, healed, and sealed the fire, and the banned has been sprouted, soaked, fermented, and cooked. Then, and only then, can they be consumed for our healthy pleasure.

My Antinutrients Tips:
- The five main "antinutrients" to remember are: phytates, lectins, gluten, tannins, and oxalates.
- Microgreens and sprouts are one of those sneaky connections, like cumin and coffee, that root from a seed and carry the same principles as nuts, seeds, grains, and legumes. For now, broccoli and kale are the microgreen/sprouts-weapons of dense nutritional choice. Eat only them. No pea shoots, amaranth, alfalfa, and all remaining associates of the seed family.

- Kale, spinach, chard, broccoli, beets, cauliflower, cabbage, onions, and any other cruciferous vegetable should be steamed before consuming because of their mild antinutrient content (oxalates) and need for being neutralized as much as possible while still maintaining important enzymes and nutrients.
- Grains, beans, and legumes are a vital part of our diet, but you need to neutralize the antinutrient content as much as possible. Once the changes have been made and the body has repaired to a point of being able to use their benefits, eat them sprouted, soaked, fermented, and cooked. Otherwise, avoid.

"What about coconut?"

Coconut anything is accepted, in small doses.

"But that's a nut!"

True, it is a nut but without the same toxic properties as the rest of the restrictions. Holding back to a maximum of 1 tablespoon of oil or butter every couple of days, if tolerable, is sufficient. Yes, coconut is an antiseptic with other benefits; it is also a diuretic and high in saturated fats. Remember: All good factors are negated by one bad. Beat the coconut-everything fad by consuming it in minimal amounts and in variety.

Unfortunately, chocolate is also off the menu. It's processed from cacao, and cacao are seeds. I always knew it but held to the tightest denial until the very end. Chocolate, and a mild silent but deadly mold issue held back my progression for months.

My Molds and Mildew Tips: Test your space for mold, fungus, and any spores that release harmful toxins. If they are obvious, treat with vinegar, hydrogen peroxide, or a vinegar and baking soda mix (paste). It's tough to believe, but they are just as effective at killing the spores as bleach and any other cleverly marketed product. Once removed, keep the area as dry as possible. These spores feed and grow from moisture.

"What do I do about getting fiber?"

Fiber may seem like a tough one because most fiber-rich foods are nuts, beans, and seeds (phytates and lectins). Nonetheless, here is a list of my approved foods that will give us our daily recommended amounts. Also, in general, the darker the color of the vegetable, the richer the fiber content. The gram measurement (g) given after each food refers to the grams of fiber in a 1-cup serving of that food.

MY SIMPLE HIGH FIBER FOODS LIST
Serving Size
1 cup
Daily Goal
A total of 25 to 50 grams of fiber spread throughout the day
VEGETABLES

Acorn squash (cubed, baked) 9g	Butternut squash (baked, cubed) 7g
Artichoke 9.6g	Cauliflower (cooked) 5g
Asparagus (cooked) 4g	Collard greens (cooked) 5g
Broccoli (boiled) 5.5g	Kale (cooked) 3g
Brussels sprouts (steamed) 4g	Mustard greens (cooked) 5g
	Okra (cooked) 4g

Parsnips (raw) 7g

Pumpkin (canned) 8g

Purple sweet potato (cubes) 5g

Spinach (cooked) 4g

Sweet potato (cubes) 4g

Swiss chard (cooked) 4g

Jackfruit (cooked) 6g

FRUITS

Avocado (1/4 medium) 3.5g

Bananas (7- to 8-inch) 3.5g

Guava (1/2 cup) 4.5g

Jackfruit (canned in water) 3g

Oranges (pieces) 4.5g

Pomegranate 6g

Raspberries 8g

"Juicing and smoothies are a great way to provide relief by adding easier to digest nutrients, when tolerated."

So says every random website in the world providing advice about the gut without ever having experienced the symptoms. The "copy and paste" method for search engine optimization. Digging deeper into the "when tolerated" includes changes made around the exact fungus, infection, and condition the body lives with and may heal from by eliminating fructose or sugar entirely or for periods of time.

Our average diet consists of nearly 3.5 ounces of sugar a day, bringing us to another much-needed change.

My Sugar Intake Recommendations

- No more than ½ ounce of sugar a day. That's one piece, or cup, of whole fruit or less a day, depending on symptoms.
- Avoid all sweeteners other than small amounts of coconut butter and fruit.

- Stick with whole low-glycemic fruits and vegetables while working through the healing. Low sugar, low starch, no seeds or skins.

Issues with bloating, gas, cramps, burning sensations, and uncomfortable feelings in your lower abdomen suggest a disruption in the lower portion of your intestines and you should avoid foods that digest in that region, also known as high-FODMAP foods: Fermentable Oligo, Di-, Monosaccharides and Polyols. Here are the low- and high-FODMAP foods that pertain to our foods list. I try to stick to the low-FODMAP foods as much as possible and consume the high in the smallest amounts and not combined. Eliminate, heal, and incorporate small amounts sporadically and slowly after.

MY SIMPLE LOW-FODMAP FOODS TO *CONSUME* LIST

VEGETABLES

Bok choy	Ginger
Carrots	Lettuce
Chives	Olives
Cucumber	Turnips

FRUITS

Bananas	Limes
Blueberries	Oranges
Lemon	Strawberries

OTHER

All meats	Ginger tea
Coconut milk (no guar gum)	Purified water
Cranberry juice	

MY SIMPLE HIGH-FODMAP FOODS TO *AVOID* LIST

VEGETABLES

Artichokes	Celery
Asparagus	Garlic
Beetroot	Leeks
Brussels sprouts	Mushrooms
Cabbage	Onions
Cauliflower	

FRUITS

Apricots	Fruit Juices
Cherries	Peaches
Coconut water	Plums
Dried Fruit	Prunes

I still can't fully absorb certain substances, like fructose. Fructose easily ferments and prevents other minerals from absorbing. Therefore, I only consume a piece or two of fruit a day that doesn't offer my body excess fructose while I continue to heal my intestinal lining and strengthen my immune system. This is a very common issue when you have a leaky gut, ulcers, inflammation, or irritation in the intestines. For all sakes of healing, here's a list of my choices for low-glycemic approved foods for avoiding fructose.

MY SIMPLE FRUCTOSE-*FRIENDLY* FOODS LIST

FRUITS

Apricot (medium)	Cranberries (1/2 cup)
Avocado (medium)	Fig, fresh (1/2 cup)
Banana (small)	Grapefruit (1/4 cup)
Blueberries (1/4 cup)	Jackfruit (1/2 cup)
Cherries (1/4 cup)	Lemon (medium)

Lime (medium)

Nectarine (1/2 cup)

Peach (1/2 cup)

Pineapple (1/2 cup)

Plum (1/2 cup)

VEGETABLES

Beets (1/2 cup, sliced)

Carrot (1 medium)

Celery (1 stalk)

Cucumber (1 cup, diced)

Iceberg lettuce (1 cup, chopped)

Mushrooms (1 cup)

Okra (1/2 cup)

Radish (1 large)

Spinach (1 cup)

Sweet potato (1/2 cup, baked)

For the first couple weeks of this process, the goal is three-quarters liquid to one-quarter solid. That means incorporating bone or vegetable broth. The bone broth provides protein and other nutrients that soothe the intestinal tract and help repair cell lining. How do you balance the remainder of the 3:1 goal? A smoothie is one way. A four- to five-ingredient, 8- to 12-ounce smoothie, blended with the variety of veggies the day needs. It's a perfect way to add more fiber, protein, and leafy greens while making it easy for the gut to digest. Nix the preprogrammed concentrated fruit juice routine. Fruit juice is terrible on the gut, providing excessive amounts of sugar, the more ounces the pour.

Here's a smoothie recipe I make often.

MEAL #3: Pineapple Ginger Smoothie

Ingredients

¼ cup pineapple chunks

1 (1-inch) piece cucumber (peeled)

½ cup bone broth

½ cup chopped collard greens

Lemon

1 (1-inch) piece ginger

Ground cinnamon

Ground turmeric

Ice, purified water

Instructions

Stick all ingredients in a to-go style blender.

Blend until creamy.

If time doesn't allow you to prepare a lunch or smoothie, combat temptations by knowing the places around you that provide the best options. The less planning, the more justification finds its appeal. Search and claw for organic, from a place that explains their practices. Avoid anything out of its natural state. This sounded so obvious for decades, until understanding that virtually nowhere puts that understanding into the food we order. Another strategy of mine is to bring half of the items for lunch, knowing the other half is easily available. However you have to do it, do it. The food and solutions are out there, and it's up to you and the pride you take in yourself to make sure they are explored to the fullest extent, without relapse. Always feel free to check the updated EWG.org clean and dirty eats list.

When I had my appendix-bursting pain, it exploded from eating a bag of raw broccoli and ranch. *"Uncle Brandon, what's in ranch?"* Deliciousness? Maybe. Immune-system inhibitors and progress zappers? Most certainly.

"But isn't broccoli good for us?"

This is true, until the gut is worn of bacteria, crawling with infections, and/or severely depleted of essential digestive enzymes and stomach acids that break down food. Missing any one allows a raw vegetable, like broccoli, to blow irritation out of proportion. The same happened from drinking milk in college during my "dehydration episodes." The same happened with coffee as the abscess was taking over. The same happened from my lunch of tomato-based chili that led to bowel resection surgery. Other foods may cause irritations, but these substances fire the shots to start a war.

From the beginning of healing and on, the goal is liquids for rest and repair, mixed with lightly sautéed, steamed, or baked veggies for easier digestion. Slowly work in more raw foods as your gut strength builds. For now, minimize raw food consumption.

"What about citrus for an acidic body?"

Citrus fruits are good. Our standard diet rich in low-quality dairy, meat, sugar, and toxins promotes acidic environments throughout the digestive tract. Citrus fruits assist with balancing the body's pH levels. Proper pH and balanced stomach acids create an environment that cancer cells cannot survive in.

It took years of commitment to spreading the truthful word for the masses to understand GMOs. They came into existence in the early 1990s and were finally required to be identified on labels in the early parts of this century's second decade. Roughly twenty years of exposure. Sadly, chemicals like Roundup go back decades before GMOs. The connection between the two? The genetically modified seeds created to be resistant to Roundup. A double dose of autoimmunity in one.

Watch the Trends and the Facts: While writing this chapter, Roundup was ordered to pay a man hundreds of millions of dollars for causing his terminal cancer. We all subconsciously (or consciously) knew that chemicals like Roundup were wearing us and our crops' quality to the point of sickness. Nevertheless, accepting it universally takes a louder voice and time's exposure. Remove from the experiment until proven healthy.

"Oh, you have an autoimmune disorder. So, you're vegan?"

A common misconception and blind correlation. Vegans protect animals and their derivatives by not consuming them. My Simple Changes avoids allergens and toxins while incorporating healers and calmers to repair and rebuild. I do not think we should treat animals the way that we do for mass production. But I do believe in eating the ones that cause the least impact on my health and the environment, only in proportion to healing. Me (and you), the earth, animals, and our sustainable ecosystem matter. Keeping our toxic load down, respecting what lives around us, minimizing our impact, and incorporating the best diet and lifestyle suitable to our healthiest survival, are what I stand by. So, to answer the question of being vegan? Meat, no. Every other animal derivative, yes.

The toxins in the soil, the feed, the medicine, the processing, and the logistics that take a newborn animal to the point of being digested are all factors that need to be considered and changed. Grass-fed meat, from animals humanely raised on good soil, like our great-grandparents' cattle used to provide all winter, is the only option. Besides removing toxin exposure, we also get denser amounts of nutrition and higher concentrations of beneficial omega fats and amino acids that are vital for the repair of tissue and gut lining. They are found in the most natural forms of certain animal meats, which is why grass-fed beef collagen is a part of the method. Nonetheless, going out and biting into our culture's accepted habit of eating a 24-ounce steak with every meal is overindulgence. Stick to 4- to 8-ounce servings, cooked for flavor and not at every meal.

Meat is important to heal the gut but not vital after the body can tolerate sprouted, soaked, and cooked grains and legumes. In order to get to that point, the antinutrients have to go or the digestive tract will never heal to where we can actually tolerate them again. Lastly, if the meat doesn't contain the lowest fat and isn't the highest quality, it's not worth the regression. Each week I roughly stick to this guideline: One, maybe two, meals with red meat, two or three meals with turkey, none or maybe one meal with chicken, one meal of sardines or salmon from a brand that tests for heavy metal toxicity or comes from a cold-water region of the world that toxic pollution hasn't affected (good luck), none to one meal of pork (only if it's a clean version of a lean loin), lamb and wild game like bison on occasional rotation, and a serving or two of beef liver. The other organs are acceptable as well. Just not for me. The reason to eat the organs are because they contain dense amounts of essential nutrients that are so often depleted in our deprived bodies. B vitamins, copper, and iron, for example, are common deficiencies with any intestinal disorder that flushes more than it absorbs, especially Crohn's disease. The taste may be less than desirable, which means marinating it in lime juice, coconut aminos, or coconut milk is recommended. The benefit is in repairing and healing. Lastly, on the seventh day of the week I give everything a break and go "meatless." Jackfruit (not in brine) is a great meat alternative with a high concentration of beneficial fiber.

With a goal of consuming 30–40 percent of your body weight in grams of protein per day (or 10 percent of your daily calorie intake, depending on levels of exercise), here are the foods I go by to make sure I am consuming enough protein to repair. (Do consult a dietitian or trainer if you're exercising more than I recommend.) The gram measurement (g) given after each vegetable, fruit or legume refers to the grams of protein in a 1-cup serving and for all meat listed refers to the grams of protein in a 4 oz per serving.

MY SIMPLE PROTEIN FOODS LIST

Serving

1 cup or 4 oz

Daily Goal

Total of 30–40 percent of your body weight in grams of protein per day

VEGETABLES

Artichoke (steamed) 4g

Arugula (raw) 3g

Asparagus (lightly sautéed) 3g

Bamboo shoots (1/2" slices, raw) 4g

Beet greens (sautéed) 3.5g

Bok choy (cooked) 4.5g

Broccoli (steamed) 4g

Brussels sprouts (steamed) 4.5g

Butternut squash (baked) 2g

Cauliflower (steamed) 2g

Collard greens (sautéed) 5g

Garlic (raw, 5 cloves) 1g

Hubbard squash (baked) 5g

Kale (sautéed) 2.5g

Leeks (raw) 4g

Okra (raw) 2g

Portabella mushrooms (grilled) 4g

Seaweed (kelp) 2g

Shiitake mushrooms (stir-fried) 3.5g

Spinach (steamed) 5g

Turnip greens (sautéed) 4.5g

Vine leaf (steamed) 4.5g

White mushrooms (boiled) 3.5g

FRUITS

Apricots 2.2g

Avocado 3g

Bananas (sliced) 1.3g

Blackberries 2g

Kiwifruit 2.1g

Oranges 2g

Peaches 1.5g

Raspberries 1.5g

MEATS (Grass fed & pasture raised)

Bison 24g

Chicken 33g

New York strip (fat trimmed) 24g

Rib-eye (fat trimmed) 23g

Filet mignon 28g

Lamb (lean loin) 25g

Ostrich 33g

Pork tenderloin or chop 25g

Turkey breast (baked) 30g

Venison 27g

BROTH (Organic)

Grass-fed beef bone broth 9g

Pasture-raised chicken bone broth 9g

Pasture-raised turkey bone broth 9g

FISH

Canned smoked sardines 23g

Wild pink salmon (cooked) 28g

"But how do I know I am getting the highest quality meat?"

Find a grocery store that uses an animal welfare rating from an independent source that verifies the animals' lifestyle and conditions. Or a butcher or farmer you trust isn't just trying to sell you their BS to make a buck.

"Oh, some of that expensive healthy foo foo food?"

Ah, the classic perception that eating healthy is expensive. So is overindulging in low-quality restaurant or store food, then paying every medical dollar it wears the body down to. My asthma inhaler was $50 each refill, with insurance. The instructions read, 2 to 4 puffs a day and see my PCP every four months for another prescription. For years I used about one inhaler a month. Total: $600 a year, for just one medication. Including the checkups, other allergy medicine, Crohn's cocktails, pain meds, nausea fixes, Xanax, antibiotics, tests, and procedures, there were grocery bills far greater than the 20 cents saved by buying a nonorganic cucumber.

Luckily, those ten asthma puffs a week have vanished as the gut inflammation subsided. No more machine. No more steroids. Or disks. Or late-night ER visits. My inhaler has been nearly empty and lost for over six months now and that helpless, fish out of the water feeling is now left in the mind of a time versions ago. That $600 gets put right into the already tight food budget.

When finally making it home after the work day, I try and greet something I love. The truth behind coming home to something you love is, when we feel securely attached with another form of life (preferably more than plants), our stress levels lower. A simple greeting of positivity reduces cortisol and adrenaline levels a little bit more. Even if your honey is a dog or cat, create the greeting. Then, shed those exhausted work clothes and change into your version of sweats and a hoodie.

This time of day, a couple of hours since that smoothie, is a perfect opportunity for a deep stretch followed by a workout. Recapping from the "Exercise" chapter:

My Exercise Plan

- Stretching: twenty to thirty minutes and slow
- Yoga, two to four times a week
- Meditation, two times a day and each at least ten minutes
- Thirty to sixty minutes of nonstrenuous, gut-fulfilling exercise. (And this doesn't mean those "cancel walks" to frozen treats and happy hour libations. Alcohol is replaced by delicious mocktails until healing proves otherwise.) A walk, hike, bike ride, lifting weights, shooting baskets, whatever gives you the release and rebalance while working the body out.
- During exercise, fluids are vital. If I am doing calisthenics, I drink purified water. If I am lifting weights, I will often incorporate a scoop of collagen peptides to the water.

It doesn't matter what combination makes up your day. Just as long as it does. Being consciously active with every day is the Simple Change.

"When do you take supplements, what supplements do you take, and what do they even do?"

This is a common question I get. Here's an easy parallel to help remember.

My Supplement Guide

- Vitamin C provides aid for getting supplies (nutrients) through the battlefield walls successfully (absorption) then assists with repairing the retaken land (digestive tract) and regenerate the walls (tissue). In the beginning phases I used vitamin C often. After things calmed, I went without it. Remember, quality and capitalism also apply to supplements.

- Turmeric (with black pepper) and fish oils provide relief for battlefield fires (inflammation).

- Digestive enzymes provide extra hands in the factories (stomach) to break down the supplies (food) that better equip troops (bacteria) for battle and make it easier to transport to the front lines (intestines).

- Probiotics bring reinforcement soldiers (good bacteria) to the front lines (intestines) and provide a healthy repopulation of bacteria inhabitants for the retaken land (the digestive tract and exposed disease portions).

- Liquid vitamin D serves as a communication connection for the repairing of processes throughout the operation (cell to cell communication). Without vitamin D's sufficient attributes, vital substances wouldn't be able to talk to, reach, and supply other processes of the body. The slightest deficiency makes each location vulnerable to an always attacking enemy.

- Liquid vitamin B reconstructs the ravaged structure (cell walls) once occupied by the opposition (bad bacteria, yeasts, fungus, parasites, etc.).
- L-glutamine and collagen restructure the structures (cells) by connecting the crumbled city walls (joining two cells for healing).

My Current Supplement Pattern: First thing I would recommend is guidance from your A-team with respect to your condition. After establishing that, this is the supplement plan I currently follow to maintain and continue to heal.

- Every day: digestive enzyme & probiotic
- Every few days: turmeric (w/black pepper) capsule
- Once a week: liquid vitamin D
- Once in a while: fish oil capsule
- Not anymore: vitamin C
- Depending on exercise: collagen, one or two scoops a day

As with any product, quality is key. Pill casings made with low-quality ingredients, liquids mixed with preservatives, and powders laced with antiaging substances are other sneaky changes. Look for no added extras, vegetable capsules, and the highest quality from minimal processing. The FDA doesn't step in unless the manufacturer claims that it can cure a disease or if the product makes people sick. Meaning, we are the experiment until proven otherwise.

Here is an example of a dinner recipe I would fix shortly after a workout, planned to balance nutrition for the day of meals.

MEAL #4: Oven Roasted Turkey (or Chicken) Breast

Following the My Simple Change we've already made: highest quality meat, and if you can't find it, then it's not worth the reset of progress.

Ingredients

1 cup sliced carrots

1 medium onion, roughly chopped (if tolerated)

Unrefined, unfiltered extra-virgin olive oil

Juice of 1 lemon

¼ cup bone broth (check ingredients and make sure they follow the recommended list for your condition)

1 turkey breast (about 1.5 pounds)

Ground turmeric

Dried tarragon

Ground ginger

Ground sage

1 medium butternut squash, halved and seeds removed

½ cup broccoli florets

1 cup arugula (or any leafy green of choice. Arugula raw, everything else steamed or sautéed)

4 to 6 black olives, sliced

¼ avocado, sliced

1 (1-inch) piece cucumber, peeled and diced

1 scallion, green part only, chopped

¼ cup sauerkraut or kimchi (or any fermented food of choice containing only cabbage, purified water, and sea salt. Maybe ginger or another whole food from the list. Otherwise, no go.)

213

Kale microgreens (amount you desire)

Instructions

Preheat the oven to 425°F for turkey (375°F for chicken).

Line the bottom of a glass baking dish with the carrots, onion, 1 tablespoon of olive oil, and the bone broth (if cooking chicken, omit bone broth).

Peel back the turkey breast skin (keeping it attached on one side) and baste with olive oil and half the lemon juice. Then, rub with turmeric, tarragon, ginger, and sage and recover with the attached skin.

Baste the butternut squash with olive oil and some turmeric and place cut-side down on a foil-lined baking sheet.

Cover the turkey with foil and place in the oven (on the same rack) with the butternut squash.

Immediately turn the temperature down to 375°F.

Bake for 45 minutes, or until the internal temperature of the breast reaches 165°F (check in the center of the thickest part of the breast) and the squash is soft when poked with a fork.

Note: If cooking chicken, baste and rub in liquid and spices, and place in the oven at 375°F for 45 minutes.

Steam the broccoli until soft, 4 to 5 minutes.

In a bowl, combine the arugula, olives, 1 tablespoon of olive oil, avocado, remaining lemon juice, cucumber, and scallion.

When the turkey and squash have finished baking, remove and allow to rest for 10 to 15 minutes.

Cut each baked squash half in two, plate one piece and store the rest in a glass container. Slice the turkey, divide into four portions, plate one and store the rest in a separate glass container.

Plate the salad, roasted veggies, and steamed broccoli. Top with the sauerkraut and microgreens.

Enjoy a simple meal that pushes nutrition forward while keeping the same flavors we love!

This last meal of the day is the most delicate. The last chance to feed and relieve digestion for the sleeping hours while providing nutrition to keep the healing train rolling forward.

"Wait, what about dessert?"

I debated back and forth about including dessert, and ultimately chose not to. Knowing how difficult it is to get a dessert that falls in line with the routine and doesn't ruin the day's progress, it's a door that needs to remain shut. Even if a sweet makes its way in, it shouldn't be the last food consumed in the day. After a day of what we just accomplished, we're going to ruin it with sugar just before going to bed? That logic puts every day on repeat.

The good things about finishing dinner before 8 p.m. and retiring early are that our digestion can process before rest and there's still more time in the day, for us. The calls, the talks, the quiet, the expansion. If there's a Change in the day that has yet to be fulfilled, now would be a good time.

"That's because I always saw Grandpa with his pipe."

If your dessert is served with nicotine, it's time to give it up. If it's enjoyed with a relaxing dose of marijuana, remember, it falls victim to the same principles Adam Smith laid out with capitalism. As development expands, and all of the strains get their names, so does exposure to sprayed toxins, molds, and loss of quality. Any plant we roll and smoke may provide the "take me away" high, but unfortunately, the other substances in the plants' buds weaken and expose the low when inhaled. Smoking is never good. Whether we're buying organic marijuana or an enhanced product through unnatural chemicals and substances, we're still inhaling toxins.

Finishing My Day: Winding everything down to the last Changes of the day. Fix the hot water or tea, wash the face, brush the teeth, and breathe. Find one more meditation. Reach for one more stretch. Embrace one more day forward. Living it like we deserve until that last note plays.

CHAPTER 13: One Lasting Sentence

September 2018

Procedure:

Endoscopy

Findings:

Normal appearing esophagus, gastric cardia and fundus.

Procedure:

CT Enterorrhaphy without and with contrast

Findings:

The stomach is well-distended and normal. No other areas of wall thickening are identified. The bowel is otherwise normal. There is no evidence of obstruction. The colon is within normal limits. No areas of active inflammation identified. Postsurgical change from partial resection of the terminal ileum with ileocolic anastomosis. Otherwise normal CT abdomen.

Procedure:

Colonoscopy

Findings:

1. Normal-appearing anal exam.

2. Normal-appearing rectum on retroflexed view.

3. Normal-appearing sigmoid colon, descending colon, splenic flexure, transverse colon, hepatic flexure, and ascending colon. Random biopsies were taken from throughout the colon to assess for possible Crohn's disease activity.

4. A surgical anastomotic site was noted in the right colon, appeared to be an ileocolonic anastomotic site. There was mild to moderate erythema and erosions at the surgical anastomotic site. Biopsies were taken from this area. The terminal ileum was not intubated.

Component:

C-Reactive Protein

Value:

.2

Reference Range

<0.80 MG/DL

VITAMIN D TOTAL

37 ng/mL L

Deficiency:

<20 ng/mL

I anxiously waited in his office. This time I came alone. These were my results and my next adjustment. As the GI opened the door, shook my hand, and sat down, my heart raced. He opened his folder and held a long pause as he reviewed the pages and charts.

"I went over your blood work and stool sample. Examined your stomach, intestines, and the surgical anastomotic site."

Another pause. He looked up.

"I could not find any active Crohn's disease in your body."

It had been 1,477 days since that "1 last treatment." Thirty-four years of life, and everything in between, cut the rope in that moment.

"I didn't see any infections or intestinal wall hardening. Your blood work looked normal and inflammation minimal. Whatever you're doing, keep doing it."

It had been eight years since removing my infected intestine, four since the shingles, three since the projected relapse for another surgery, and one since the last true flare-up. The nausea has subsided; hip pains have vanished; colds an afterthought; asthma diminished; burning, cramping, bile-filled stools, blood, anxiety, and pinpricking, gone. No more inhalers, allergy relievers, pain solvers, antibiotic bacteria killers, nausea reducers, anxiety calmers, or the dark place justifiers.

The Crohn's disease was finally in remission. Diet, lifestyle, and persistence resolved the unresolved. I could've easily found the answers sooner had I taken more responsibility. But that's a lesson only to be learned with time.

My hope is that understanding alone is enough to alter your course to start making the Changes. You don't deserve to suffer anymore. Not when you don't have to. Not when the Changes are this Simple, and the results can happen. I always believed that I could, justification's doubt questioned if it would, and…well, it did.

Will I get sick again? Of course. Even the healthiest get sick. But whatever does come next, whenever that may be, I will deal with it and adjust from there, building in the best routines and navigating through what's working, what my body is calling for.

This book is the least I can do to hopefully minimize your own days to remission and unload the gun to Russian roulette, by simply just paying it forward. It's a daunting task to travel down a road with an unclear ending. To help you more on your navigation to your solution you can find all of my suggestions for food, products, meditation and yoga videos, my videos, mental health help, recipes, news, and more on the www.MySimpleChanges.com website. Remember, we're all in this together, but it's your choice and your course.

"You'll find your way through this. Stay willing."

The two-time cancer survivor at my "1 Last Treatment" was right. She found her way through it, pushed me toward it, and now you're on your way too.

Stay willing.

INDEX

Made in the USA
Columbia, SC
25 June 2020